Synthesizing Qua

T0252142

Synthesizing Qualitative Research

Choosing the Right Approach

Edited by
Karin Hannes
Centre for Methodology of Educational Research, Faculty of Psychology and Education, K.U. Leuven; Centre for Evidence-Based Medicine-Belgian Branch of the Cochrane Collaboration, Belgium

Craig Lockwood
The Joanna Briggs Institute, Faculty of Health Sciences, The University of Adelaide, Australia

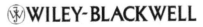

WILEY-BLACKWELL

A John Wiley & Sons, Ltd., Publication

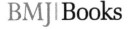

This edition first published 2012 © 2012 by John Wiley & Sons, Ltd.

BMJ Books is an imprint of BMJ Publishing Group Limited, used under licence by Blackwell Publishing which was acquired by John Wiley & Sons in February 2007. Blackwell's publishing programme has been merged with Wiley's global Scientific, Technical and Medical business to form Wiley-Blackwell.

Registered office: John Wiley & Sons, Ltd, The Atrium, Southern Gate, Chichester, West Sussex, PO19 8SQ, UK

Editorial offices: 9600 Garsington Road, Oxford, OX4 2DQ, UK

The Atrium, Southern Gate, Chichester, West Sussex, PO19 8SQ, UK

111 River Street, Hoboken, NJ 07030-5774, USA

For details of our global editorial offices, for customer services and for information about how to apply for permission to reuse the copyright material in this book please see our website at www.wiley.com/wiley-blackwell

The right of the author to be identified as the author of this work has been asserted in accordance with the UK Copyright, Designs and Patents Act 1988.

Library of Congress Cataloging-in-Publication Data

Synthesizing qualitative research : choosing the right approach / edited by Karin Hannes, Craig Lockwood.

p. ; cm.

Includes bibliographical references and index.

ISBN 978-0-470-65638-9 (pbk.)

1. Qualitative research. 2. Medicine–Research–Methodology. 3. Biology–Research–Methodology.

I. Hannes, Karin. II. Lockwood, Craig, 1971-

[DNLM: 1. Qualitative Research. 2. Biomedical Research–methods. 3. Meta-Analysis as Topic. W 20.5]

R853.Q34S96 2011

610.72′1–dc23   2011022676

A catalogue record for this book is available from the British Library.

This book is published in the following electronic formats: ePDF 9781119959816; Wiley Online Library 9781119959847; ePub 9781119959823

Set in 9.5/12pt Minion by Thomson Digital, Noida, India

1   2012

This book is dedicated to the future of synthesis science; a disparate field with rich potential for further methodological development. We trust that this book makes both a useful, practical contribution to what is known here and now and enables the next generation of students, academics, theorists, and researchers to draw upon some of today's best synthesis scientists for tomorrow's methodology.

Contents

List of contributors

Nicky Britten, PhD
Professor of Applied Health Care Research
Peninsula Medical School
University of Exeter
Exeter, Devon, UK

Fiona Campbell
Research Associate
School of Health and Related Research
University of Sheffield
Sheffield, UK

Jamie L. Crandell, PhD
Research Assistant Professor
University of North Carolina at Chapel Hill, NC
USA

Kate Flemming, PhD RN
Research Fellow
Department of Health Sciences
The University of York
York, UK

Karin Hannes, PhD
Doctor-Assistant
Centre for Methodology of Educational Research
Faculty of Psychology and Education, K.U.Leuven
Belgium

Centre for Evidence-Based Medicine
Belgian Branch of the Cochrane Collaboration
Belgium

Angela Harden, PhD
Professor of Community and Family Health
Institute for Health and Human Development
School of Health and Biosciences
University of East London
London, UK

Josephine Kavanagh, BA, MA
Research Officer
EPPI-Centre
Social Science Research Unit
Institute of Education
University of London
London, UK

Nathan Manning, PhD
Systematic Reviewer
Kleijnen Systematic Reviews and Adjunct Research Fellow
The Joanna Briggs Institute
The University of Adelaide
Australia

Elizabeth McInnes, PhD
Deputy Director
Nursing Research Institute – Australian Catholic University and St Vincents
and Mater Health Sydney
National Centre for Clinical Outcomes Research (NaCCOR)
St Vincent's Hospital
Darlinghurst, NSW
Australia

Barbara L. Paterson, RN PhD
Professor & Dean
Thompson Rivers University
School of Nursing
Kamloops BC
Canada

Catherine Pope, PhD
Professor of Medical Sociology
University of Southampton
Southampton, UK

Alan Pearson, AM
Executive Director
The Joanna Briggs Institute
Faculty of Health Sciences
University of Adelaide
Australia

Margarete Sandelowski, PhD RN
Cary C. Boshamer Distinguished Professor
University of North Carolina at Chapel Hill
Chapel Hill, NC
USA

James Thomas, PhD
Reader in Social Policy
EPPI-Centre
Social Science Research Unit
Institute of Education
University of London
London, UK

Corrine I. Voils, PhD
Associate Professor of Medicine
Durham Veterans Affairs Medical Center and Duke
University Medical Center
Durham, NC
USA

Geoff Wong, MD(Res)
Senior Lecturer in Primary Health Care and GP Principal
Healthcare Innovation and Policy Unit
Centre for Health Sciences
Blizard Institute
Barts and The London School of Medicine and Dentistry
London, UK

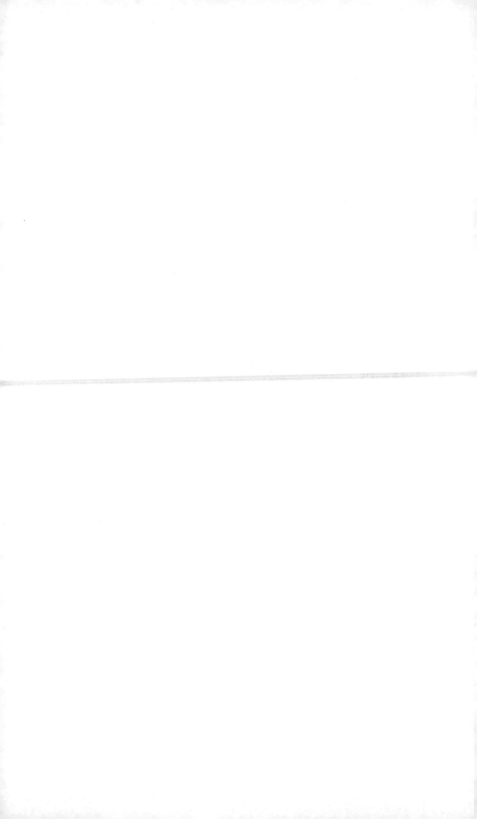

Preface

The growth in qualitative evidence synthesis methods, and the increasing number of reviews that are published using these methods, is a clear indicator that what was once a field for the "interested few" is becoming mainstream practice. There are now large numbers of published qualitative synthesis papers, as well as a growing body of academic and theoretical work to further inform the conduct of qualitative reviews, and to further stimulate methodological development. It is within the last few years that the majority of methodological development has occurred, and within this timeframe, good theorists have enhanced and refined their methods, as is evident in the quality of published qualitative synthesis reports seen in mainstream journals to date. The majority of methodological guidance though is buried in websites or published in specialized journals. The few books available tend to have a limited focus on a particular methodology, or are theoretical rather than practical. Methodology papers in journals serve to flag issues or ideas, but limitations prevent the level of depth and explanation possible in a book. The word limit of journal articles prevents many authors from comprehensively describing their full methods, and providing appropriate illustration or exemplars is also problematic in most journals.

Writing about synthesis methods included the process of choosing between different approaches, selecting what would be appropriate for this particular book and what would be put into the drawer until a new opportunity for writing arose. Although first intended as a compendium of all qualitative evidence synthesis methods, we decided to focus this book on six commonly used methodologies for qualitative evidence synthesis. We opted to portray those synthesis approaches that have particularly been developed by and for researchers involved in systematically reviewing literature. Our choice has been influenced by previously published overviews of approaches from colleague methodologists, personal knowledge, and connections and the conversations that occur in our respective fields internationally. We have focused on methods that have been developed with the aim of synthesizing primary studies, providing the reader with a detailed stepwise description on how to move from original research texts to a review of qualitative literature. We believe that these approaches will generate interest from the international community of researchers, practitioners and policymakers currently involved in qualitative evidence synthesis.

The book is meant to be a guide to reviewers and users from any discipline, although most of the worked examples are situated in the field of healthcare. It is not a penultimate book of methods for qualitative synthesis, neither will everyone agree with our particular selection and how we have categorized them. Approaches that have been used in practice but are not covered in our book include narrative summary, thematic analysis, grounded theory, meta-study, cross-case techniques, content analysis, case survey, and qualitative comparative analysis methods. Some of these methods have drawn upon the principles of basic research designs. These adapted versions of basic research methods for the purpose of synthesis are promising, but currently lack the transparency important to a community of researchers involved in systematic reviewing. They offer little guidance on particular aspects such as search strategies, critical appraisal, and sampling of primary studies, neither do they discuss why these should or should not be done. Furthermore, they lack clarity of the particular features of the synthesis approach as compared to other synthesis methods and have not yet formally been subject to an evaluation of their appropriateness in the context of systematically reviewing literature.

The methods included here are some of the better developed and used approaches available at this point in time; yet no single text has brought them together before, nor provided the diverse and high quality example syntheses that the authors, and in some chapters, originators of the methodology have conducted. Some of the synthesis methods presented are meant to build theory and deepen understanding, while others have been created to develop lines of action for policy and practice or to provide the current state of the art on a particular topic. We feel it is most important that those engaging in a qualitative or mixed method evidence synthesis have a clear understanding of what particular approaches intend to do and which method best fits a researcher's goal and epistemological position.

Most researchers publishing qualitative or mixed-method syntheses do not successfully answer the question of why, among other approaches, they have opted for a particular method. Generally authors state that their choice was influenced by what fits their particular school of thought or by what others have successfully used in the past. The latter is particularly the case for meta-ethnography, currently a very commonly used approach and one of the few that has published methodological guidance. This is a substantive limitation though which offers future reviewers limited opportunities to critique or gain insights from such decision-making processes. This book not only offers to guide readers and potential users in how to apply a particular approach, it also guides general readers through the considerations as to why they should opt to choose a certain approach for their research project. Through the presentation of worked examples of different approaches, it brings more balance and a more insightful perspective to the options available to researchers. The book does not simply resort to technical reporting of method, but rather focuses on illustrating the challenges users of an approach are likely to come across. These challenges are often hidden or only partly addressed in published articles, where the main interest is to present the content of the work rather than the methodology.

In summary, we believe this book provides a detailed and integrated resource for readers who would otherwise have to piece together methodology from a disparate range of journal articles and other resources. We do not see this book as an end point, since much remains to be learned and written within the field of qualitative and mixed-method synthesis. Instead, we hope to stimulate further pragmatic, intellectual, and methodological curiosity in the richly rewarding field of qualitative evidence synthesis.

Karin Hannes
Craig Lockwood

Acknowledgements

We would not do justice to the hard work of the contributing authors on each of their worked examples, if we were not to put them first on our list of people to acknowledge. For some of them the production of their chapters coincided with serious life events, including very positive experiences but also more challenging issues, on a personal or a professional level. Therefore, a special thank you for the commitment and dedication that finally led us to the publication of this book is appropriate. We sincerely thank all academics that have assisted us in completing the initial peer review of the included chapters; Wim Van den Noortgate, Patrick Onghena and Mieke Heyvaert from the Centre for Methodology of Educational Research at K.U. Leuven, and Nathan Manning, former employee of the Joanna Briggs Institute. We also thank the staff members from both our hosting institutes for enthusiastically following up on the progress of the book. In addition, conversations and debates on approaches to qualitative evidence synthesis with methodological experts worldwide and colleague researchers from other research institutes have inspired us to embark on this particular journey, not least the Cochrane Qualitative Research Methods Group, whose convenors have been a wonderful forum for discussion and truly enriched our understanding of evidence synthesis.

We are most grateful for permission given to reproduce extracts from the following:

Figure 2.1 Reproduced with permission from the Joanna Briggs Institute, Reviewers' Manual, 2008.

Figures 2.3 to 2.6 Reproduced from Hannes K, Goedhuys J & Aertgeerts B. Obstacles to implementing Evidence-Based Practice in Belgium: a context-specific qualitative evidence synthesis including findings from different health care disciplines. *Acta Clinica Belgica* (in press), with permission from Acta Clinica Belgica.

Figures 3.1 and 3.2 Reproduced from Pound *et al.* Resisting Medicines: a synthesis of qualitative studies of medicine taking. *Social Science & Medicine* 2005; **61**(1): 133–155, 2005, with permission from Elsevier.

Figure 4.1 and Tables 4.2, 4.4 and 4.5 Reproduced from Flemming K. 'Synthesis of quantitative and qualitative research: an example using Critical Interpretive Synthesis', Journal of Advanced Nursing 2010; 66(1):201–217, 2010, with permission from John Wiley & Sons Ltd.

Table 4.3 Reproduced from Flemming K. 'Synthesis of quantitative and qualitative research: an example using Critical Interpretive Synthesis', Journal of Advanced Nursing 2010; 66(1):201–217, 2010, (using data from Hawker *et al* 2002), with permission from John Wiley & Sons Ltd.

Figure 6.1 Reproduced from Harden A, Garcia J, Oliver S, Rees R, Shepherd J, Brunton G, Oakley A, Applying systematic review methods to studies of people's views: an example from public health, *Journal of Epidemiology and Community Health* **58**: 794–800, 2004, with permission from BMJ Publishing Group Ltd.

Figure 6.2 Reproduced from Campbell F, Johnson M, Messina J, *et al.* Behavioural interventions for weight management in pregnancy: A systematic review of quantitative and qualitative data. *BMC Public Health* 2011, **11**:491 doi:10.1186/1471–2458–11–491

Table 7.1 and Figure 7.1 Adapted from Voils *et al.* 2009 with permission from the Royal Society of Medicine Press, London.

Chapter 1 "It looks great but how do I know if it fits?": an introduction to meta-synthesis research

Barbara L. Paterson, RN PhD

Thompson Rivers University, School of Nursing, Kamloops BC, Canada

In the past decade, there has been a proliferation of methods to synthesize qualitative research studies. Although several qualitative evidence synthesis methods share common epistemological tenets, developers of these methods rarely make clear how their particular method differs from and is unique to other synthesis records. The following chapter is intended both as an introduction to the book and as a way of making sense of the multiple epistemological, theoretical, and methodological interpretations of qualitative evidence synthesis that are apparent in the synthesis methods that exist today. The chapter provides a general overview of the history and current state-of-the-art of qualitative evidence synthesis. It also includes a general overview of qualitative evidence synthesis methods and a framework to assist researchers in the selection of a synthesis method.

Introduction

Qualitative evidence synthesis, the focus of this book, is defined as the study of qualitative studies (Patterson *et al.* 2001). It is the synthesis or amalgamation of individual qualitative research reports (commonly called "primary research reports") that relate to a specific topic or focus in order to arrive at new or enhanced understanding about the phenomenon under study. It entails an interpretive process by which "the constituent study texts can be treated as the multivocal interpretation of a phenomenon, just as the voices of different participants might be in a single qualitative study" (Zimmer 2006). In the 1990s there existed few definitive guidelines about how qualitative evidence synthesis could be enacted. Now, a decade later, almost every journal

Synthesizing Qualitative Research: Choosing the Right Approach, First Edition.
Edited by Karin Hannes and Craig Lockwood.
© 2012 John Wiley & Sons, Ltd. Published 2012 by John Wiley & Sons, Ltd.

in the health and social sciences contains articles about the need for qualitative synthesis to provide evidence to support clinical practice and to identify directions for future research.

There has been a proliferation of ideas about how to conduct qualitative synthesis, each set of authors offering different insights about how this could be best achieved, and most suggesting that their method is the most credible. However, there exists much confusion about how the various synthesis methods compare to each other and the factors that researchers should consider to determine which method best suits their needs, purposes, and ideological stance. This chapter is intended both as an introduction to the book and as a way of making sense of the multiple qualitative evidence synthesis methods that exist. The chapter consists of a brief overview of the uses and evolution of qualitative evidence synthesis methods, including how the various synthesis methods compare to one another. Following this synopsis, I will detail the factors that researchers should consider when selecting particular qualitative evidence synthesis methods. In conclusion, I will provide an overview of the contributions of the book to the field of qualitative evidence synthesis.

The uses of qualitative evidence synthesis

The appeal of qualitative evidence synthesis lies mainly in its ability to effect outcomes that are not feasible or possible in a single qualitative study. By providing a broad overview of a body of qualitative research, syntheses can reveal more powerful explanations that are available in a single study, leading to greater generalizability of the research findings and often to increased levels of abstraction (Sherwood 1999). A synthesis of multiple qualitative studies can also refute or revise the current understanding of a particular phenomenon. For example, a synthesis of qualitative research about the experience of living with a chronic illness (Paterson 2001) resulted in a model of chronic illness that challenged the current notions about the trajectory of chronic illness as linear with one ideal end-point. In addition, qualitative evidence synthesis can assist researches to: explore differences and similarities across settings, sample populations, and researchers' disciplinary, methodological and/or theoretical perspectives (NHS CRD 2001); generate operational models, theories, or hypotheses that can be tested in later research (Thorne & Paterson 1998); identify gaps and areas of ambiguity in the body of research, thereby revealing directions for future research (NHS CRD 2001); provide a historical overview of the development of concepts or theories over time (Paterson *et al.* 2001); complement the findings or the interpretation of quantitative systematic reviews (Tranfield 2006); and inform the development of questionnaires or surveys by identifying the significant attributes of a phenomenon (Tranfield 2006).

The origins of qualitative evidence synthesis

There is some debate as to where the idea of qualitative synthesis first originated. Walsh and Downe (2005) indicate that Stern and Harris were the first to refer to the need for qualitative evidence synthesis, while Paterson and colleagues (2001) acknowledge the work of Statham, Mauksch, and Miller as pioneering this concept. It is generally agreed, however, that the need for a comparative analysis of the findings of qualitative research was stimulated by the explosion of single qualitative research studies in the 1980s and 1990s.

As early as 1997, Sandelowski, Docerty, and Emden (1997) cautioned qualitative researchers that they were in danger of "eternally reinventing the wheel" unless they found some way of identifying and categorizing the relationships between findings of various qualitative studies. At the same time there was growing recognition of the need to use empirical evidence to inform policy and practice (Garrett & Thomas 2004). Researchers began to entertain the notion that qualitative research could be synthesized to contribute evidence to the field. In the quantitative research realm, the method of *meta-analysis*[1] (Glass *et al.* 1981) gave rise to an increasing appreciation for the synthesis of research, particularly as published meta-analyses were shown to contribute many benefits, such as the assessment of empirical evidence and generating theory (Russell 2005). However, until recently, the world of systematic reviews has been dominated by syntheses of quantitative research using the techniques of meta-analysis. This in part reflects the reputation of qualitative research as less credible and rigoros than quantitative research (Pearson 2004). It also mirrors the competing and often conflicting understandings of what qualitative evidence synthesis is and how to enact it.

Historical overview

There have been four distinct phases in the evolution of qualitative synthesis. In the first phase in the late 1980s to the 2000s, two educational researchers, Noblit and Hare (1998), delineated the steps of qualitative evidence synthesis in their book about *"meta-ethnography."* These authors referred

---

[1] Italicized terms introduced in this chapter are defined at the conclusion of the chapter in Table 1.1.

to meta-ethnography as involving the comparison, analysis, interpretation, and translation of the findings of individual qualitative studies. Although the method has undergone some recent adaptations, it continues to be one of the most popular synthesis methods.

The second phase in the development of qualitative evidence synthesis methods was the introduction of *meta-study* (2001) in the early 2000s. Meta-study is in keeping with the interpretive paradigm (2001); consequently, this method emphasizes qualitative evidence synthesis as an interpretive process. The developers of this method argue that because qualitative research focuses on meaning *in context*, a synthesis of qualitative research studies must capture how the sociocultural and historical context of the primary research, as well as the research method and theoretical frames of such research, influenced what questions the qualitative researchers asked, their research design, and their interpretation of the data (2001).

The third phase of the evolution of qualitative evidence synthesis in the years following the publication of the text on meta-study is characterized by the inclusion of qualitative research in systematic reviews. The Cochrane Collaboration, which had previously relied exclusively on the results of quantitative studies, developed a Qualitative Methods Group to develop and disseminate methods for incorporating qualitative evidence in *systematic reviews* (Booth 2001). Developers of qualitative synthesis methods that purport to conduct a systematic review commonly typify the Cochrane Collaboration in their understanding of such a review as both systematic and rigoros. They emphasize that if the findings of qualitative syntheses are to be seen as credible and trustworthy, qualitative research syntheses must include a critical and transparent appraisal of the research (Pearson 2004). Such researchers have developed critical appraisal tools and computer data analysis software (e.g., Qualitative Assessment and Review Instrument) for such purposes (McInnes & Wimpenny 2008).

The fourth phase in the history of qualitative evidence synthesis has occurred simultaneously with the third phase. Synthesis methods introduced in this phase focus on integrating qualitative and quantitative research in the following ways: (1) using quantitative meta-analysis and statistical techniques to quantify the impact, quality, and/or relevance of the findings of primary research studies; (2) using qualitative interpretive methods to identify prevalent themes in the quantitative and qualitative research within a body of research; and (3) combining the results of an aggregation of the findings of quantitative research with that of qualitative research and then using quantitative and/or qualitative strategies to synthesize or determine the weight of the evidence of this aggregated data. An example of a combined qualitative–quantitative synthesis is the work of Thomas and colleagues

(Thomas *et al.* 2003) in identifying interventions that promote children's intake of fruits and vegetables. The researchers conducted a meta-analysis of quantitative studies and a *thematic analysis* of qualitative research. Then they developed a matrix to show how effective interventions were connected to children's views about those interventions.

Several researchers (e.g., Sandelowski, Thorne, Noblit) who initially pioneered synthesis methods have evolved in their understanding of how to conduct qualitative evidence synthesis, in part because of the increasing sophistication of understanding in the field of evidence synthesis and in part in response to what funders and other stakeholders now demand in terms of credible evidence. Sandelowski, for example, initially questioned the merit of obscuring the richness of qualitative findings by synthesizing them (Sandelowski *et al.* 1997) but recently, following her experience in synthesizing several hundred qualitative studies about women with HIV/AIDS, she has espoused the quantitative aggregative techniques of *meta-summary* in part as a means of addressing the critiques of qualitative synthesis as lacking standards of rigor and needing to account for issues of credibility and validity in qualitative syntheses (Gough & Elbourne 2002).

An overview of qualitative synthesis methods

In 2003, Finfgeld (2003) identified five various qualitative evidence synthesis methods. Since then, at least a dozen more have been developed. Despite their epistemological, methodological, and terminological differences, qualitative evidence synthesis methods share the common attributes of (1) involving a team of researchers (i.e., it is rare to encounter qualitative research syntheses that involve a lone researcher), (2) investigating a number of primary research reports, and (3) organizing the synthesis according to a concept, theory, and/or research objective (Yager 2006).

Most synthesis methods can be categorized according to where they fit in relation to specific attributes (Figure 1.1). Three of these attributes (*aggregative/interpretive*, epistemology, and degree of iteration) occur on a continuum; that is, synthesis methods can be categorized according to where they fit in a range between two poles. A defining attribute is whether the method is mainly interpretive or mainly aggregative.

Qualitative evidence synthesis methods include elements of both aggregation and interpretation, but one of these is more prominent than the other in each method. Mainly aggregative synthesis methods entail listing the findings of various primary research studies and then further combining them into themes or similar descriptors to produce a general description of the phenomenon under study; they treat the findings as if they

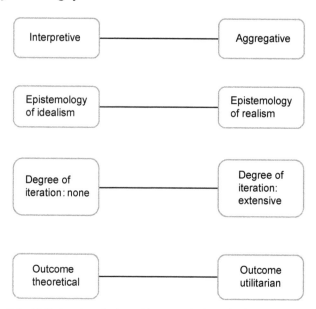

Figure 1.1   Attributes of qualitative evidence synthesis methods.

are isolated from the contexts in which they occurred. Mainly interpretive synthesis methods, on the other hand, extend the aggregation of findings to produce a new abstract model or theory of the phenomenon under study that considers the context under which the research was conducted, the data interpreted, and the research report written (Gough & Elbourne 2002). Examples of mainly aggregative methods are the systematic review method used by the Joanna Briggs Institute, meta-summary, thematic analysis, *content analysis, case survey, qualitative comparative analysis,* and *Bayesian meta-analysis* (McInnes & Wimpenny 2008). Examples of mainly interpretive methods are meta-study, *narrative synthesis, narrative summary,* formal *grounded theory,* and meta-ethnography (McInness & Wimpenny 2008).

Another attribute of synthesis methods is the epistemological position. The range of epistemological stances in qualitative evidence synthesis methods extends from idealism, wherein the researcher assumes that all knowledge is constructed, to realism in which researchers assume that they see the world as it is (Spencer *et al.* 2003). The developers of narrative synthesis (Popay *et al.* 2007), critical interpretive synthesis (CIS) (Dixon-Woods *et al.* 2006a), and meta-study (Paterson *et al.* 2001) indicate that the methods represent a 'subjective idealist' method. However, other methods (e.g., *ecological triangulation, framework synthesis, thematic synthesis*) hold to a more realist stance that highlights the possibility for research to adequately represent an external reality.

Another defining attribute of qualitative evidence synthesis methods is the degree of iteration. Some methods, such as meta-study, formal grounded theory, or thematic analysis, are iterative and circular in their processes. Researchers using these methods often revise their initial decisions and processes as they progress in the synthesis and encounter new data or reflect on the primary research. Other methods, such as framework synthesis or thematic synthesis, provide a highly structured approach to selecting, orga-nizing, and tabulating the primary research data. Qualitative evidence synthesis methods also vary as to their intended outcomes. For example, developers of thematic synthesis (Thomas *et al.* 2003; Harden *et al.* 2004; Thomas *et al.* 2007) view the intended product of such a synthesis as informing practice or policy. Kearney (2001), on the other hand, indicates that the outcome of formal grounded theory is a middle-range theory that can be tested in future research.

The defining attributes of a particular synthesis method are often inter-connected and influence one another. For example, methods that have a realist epistemological stance tend not to alter their research question or their review process during the synthesis and the primary research literature is not problematized (Yager 2006).

Making sense of the myriad of qualitative evidence synthesis methods

Despite the advances in qualitative evidence synthesis, there continues to be considerable debate within the field that centers around the various philo-sophical and methodological underpinnings of the synthesis methods and the terminology that is used. Researchers who promote a particular qualitative evidence synthesis method often admit to making adaptations to existing synthesis methods but rarely do they explicate why they made them.

It is common to see that researchers have amalgamated synthesis methods, even if the methods differ considerably in their epistemological and meth-odological underpinnings, without stating why they chose to do this. For example, Bélanger and Rodríguez (2008) state in their synthesis of qualitative research on multidisciplinary primary care teams that, "Our work has been largely inspired by the Sandelowski and Barroso" (2007) method (p. 588) but in fact, cite Paterson and colleagues' (2001) guidelines for how to analyze data using the procedures of meta-ethnography. Thorpe and colleagues (2009) indicate that their qualitative evidence synthesis drew on the methods described by Zimmer (2006), although Zimmer discussed more than one synthesis method and these had different epistemological foundations. In the past decade, there have been several efforts to address the limitations and ambiguities of the previous qualitative evidence synthesis methods.

Books have been written proposing specific synthesis methods and providing procedural steps and guidelines on how to implement those methods. Each of these texts has highlighted the complexity of qualitative evidence synthesis; they have called for qualitative researchers to continue to explore and share their insights about qualitative evidence synthesis. None, however, provide much guidance about how to determine which of the existing synthesis methods the best fit is for their purposes. I do not wish to imply that making such a decision is an easy one. Different synthesis teams make such a decision based on their unique notions of which considerations or criteria are the priority. There is also considerable overlap and ambiguity in the descriptions of many qualitative evidence synthesis methods. It may not always be clear, for example, how to determine what the anticipated outcomes of the synthesis will be. Despite these caveats, I offer the following as possible considerations when selecting the qualitative evidence synthesis method you use.

The nature of the research

Will the synthesis method result in the expected and desired outcomes?
Is the method congruent with the goals of the synthesis project?

The nature of the research includes consideration of whether the qualitative evidence synthesis method will result in the expected and desired outcomes; that is, whether the method fits the goals of the synthesis project. The outputs of synthesis methods that have a more idealist and constructivist orientation, such as meta-narrative and CIS, are generally complex and conceptual. They offer useful insights to policymakers and practitioners but require further interpretation before they can be applied to practice or policy development (Yager 2006). In contrast, realist methods, such as thematic synthesis, tend to produce outcomes that are more concrete and definitive; for example, a list of key dimensions of the phenomenon under study.

If the anticipated outcome is the development of a theory, you may consider a qualitative evidence synthesis method that promises to generate theory, such as formal grounded theory or meta-study. However, if your intention is to produce findings that will have immediate utility to informing directions for policy, you should select a method that is intended for such a purpose, such as thematic synthesis. An additional consideration is the type and quality of the primary research that is available. At times, the available primary research may be too few or too many, too homogenous or too heterogeneous, to enact the procedures of a particular synthesis method in the way the developers prescribe. For example, Wilson and Amir (2008) rejected meta-ethnography as a synthesis method when they discovered that the six primary research reports they had located were so different that they could not effectively enact the third phase of meta-ethnography, the translation of studies into one another. Although they briefly contemplated conducting the third phase within a subset of the studies, they concluded that they had too few studies to do that.

Nature of the research team

Is there the necessary mix of disciplinary, methodological, and other perspectives among the research team to enact this method?

Is the expertise needed for this method (e.g., statistical analysis, theoretical expertise) available?

In selecting a qualitative evidence synthesis method, researchers should ask themselves what the research team requires in terms of skills, knowledge, perspectives, and experiences to carry out a particular method and whether they have these. Some synthesis methods require a research team that is diverse in terms of their expertise and experience. The developers of meta-study (Paterson *et al.* 2001) indicate that this complex synthesis method requires researchers who offer different disciplinary and methodological expertise to examine a body of qualitative research. However, recently Paterson (2009) revised this measure of diversity to include variations in both academic and clinical experience. Other synthesis methods, such as that promoted by the Joanna Briggs Institute, can be carried out by two researchers who do not necessarily have content expertise in the field of study (McInnes & Wimpenny 2008). Still other synthesis methods, such as those that use quantitative strategies, for example Bayesian meta-analysis, require specific expertise, such as statistical analysis and quantitative research techniques.

Nature of the researcher

How tolerant is the researcher to the amount of structure and ambiguity that is inherent in the method?

Is his/her epistemological stance congruent with that of the synthesis method?

Researchers vary in their personal preferences regarding research methods. Some synthesis methods may appeal to some researchers but not others. Some synthesis methods are ambiguous in how they are enacted and the procedural steps are not clearly defined. This can be extremely frustrating for a novice synthesist or someone who prefers a structured method (Wilson & Amir 2008). However, McInnes and Wimpenny (2008) caution that even seemingly structured methods require some level of interpretation at the synthesis stage and this interpretation defies fixed rules. The epistemological stance of the researcher must also be considered in the selection of a qualitative research method. Researchers should select a synthesis method that best fits their view of research epistemology. Researchers whose epistemological stance supports the use of formal appraisal criteria or checklists to determine if a primary research report has sufficient quality to be included, will appreciate synthesis methods such as meta-narrative and thematic synthesis because they provide criteria on which to base exclusion and inclusion decisions. However, they are likely to be frustrated with methods that are more inclusive of primary research regardless of quality, such as meta-study and meta-ethnography (Finlayson & Dixon 2008).

Resource requirements

How much personnel, time and effort are required for this method?
Is there adequate funding to support expenses incurred in implementing this method?
Does the primary research support the method?

Qualitative evidence synthesis methods differ significantly in their resource requirements, and consequently, in their requirements for funding. The methodological complexity of a particular method should be considered in the selection decision because it will determine what resources are needed to undertake and complete a qualitative evidence synthesis. In addition, researchers proposing to conduct a qualitative evidence synthesis should also consider the number of researchers who are to be involved in the synthesis project. Synthesis methods vary in whether they can be accomplished by one or two researchers or whether they require a team of experts. Some qualitative evidence synthesis methods, such as meta-study, require considerable personnel, time, and effort; others, such as meta-ethnography, can be accomplished with a few people over a few months. If regular research team meetings and the provision for relationship building are critical to a synthesis method, such as in meta-study, researchers should consider if the available funding will cover this. Meetings of the team may entail costs of researchers' travel to attend the meetings if they do not live in the same region as the team leader, or the costs of other meeting venues such as videoconference or web-based conferences (Paterson *et al.* 2009). Some synthesis methods require funds to support the purchase of qualitative and/or quantitative data analysis software programs and funding for personnel who enter data into these programs. Others have costs related to literature retrieval and file management.

An example

In order to illustrate the selection framework described above, I will compare and contrast three synthesis methods as to their relevance and applicability to a particular synthesis project; in this case the synthesis of research about women's experience of menopause. The decision making process is illustrated in Figure 1.2. The aim of this project is to inform the practice of health practitioners regarding the care of menopausal women. The lead researcher has experience conducting grounded theory studies and has participated in two meta-ethnographies; the other researcher has recently completed a dissertation using ethnographic research methods and does not have either grounded theory or synthesis experience. Both are nurses. The researchers intend to apply for funding to conduct the synthesis from a small research grants program at their university. The three methods are critical interpretive synthesis (CIS), formal grounded theory, and thematic synthesis. I chose these methods because they represent different views of the synthesis process. With the exception of formal grounded theory they are later discussed by Flemming and Kavanagh and colleagues. As I have stated previously, there are a myriad of synthesis methods. Readers of this book will have the opportunity to explore in depth specific methods in the following chapters.

Critical interpretive synthesis is a subjective idealist method that entails a lines-of-argument synthesis in which researchers develop 'synthetic constructs' that are then linked with constructs that are found in the primary research literature (Dixon-Woods *et al.* 2006a). Formal grounded theory (Thomas *et al.* 2007) is based on an objective realist stance. Its purpose is to develop new or expanded theory about a phenomenon based on the similarities, not the differences, between the primary research reports.

Thematic synthesis is a critical realist approach to qualitative evidence synthesis that entails inductively coding and identifying analytic themes in primary research reports (Harden *et al.* 2004; Thomas *et al.* 2007).

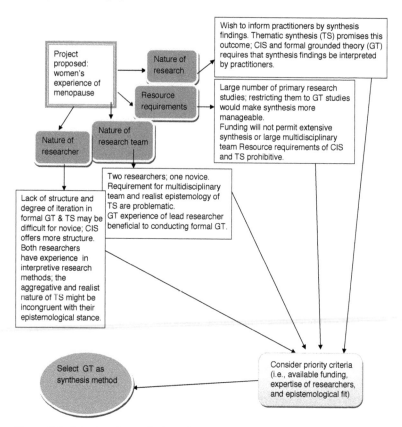

Figure 1.2 Selection of a synthesis method.

Two of the synthesis methods (CIS and thematic synthesis) are intended to elicit directives for practitioners, the purpose of the specific synthesis project; however, CIS and formal grounded theory produce a theoretical model that will require practitioners to further interpret the relevance and applicability of the synthesis findings (Dixon-Woods *et al.* 2006b). Only thematic synthesis produces findings that directly inform practitioners (Thomas & Harden 2008). The lack of structure and the degree of iteration in formal grounded theory and thematic synthesis might be challenging for the novice synthesist; CIS offers more structural guidelines for the synthesis component than the other methods. Both CIS and thematic synthesis allow for the inclusion of a variety of methods in the primary research; CIS permits the inclusion of quantitative studies in addition to the qualitative research.

Formal grounded theory is based exclusively on grounded theory studies; this may be a benefit to the synthesis project because the number of qualitative studies about menopause is huge (several hundred) and restricting the primary research to only grounded theory research will result in the project being more manageable and less costly than if there are no such restrictions. In addition, the lead researcher has experience in grounded theory but not in the other methods. If the researchers decide on another synthesis method, they will need to consider including another researcher who is more experienced in that method of synthesis.

Another consideration is that the developers of CIS place considerable emphasis on the need for a multidisciplinary team of researchers (Dixon-Woods *et al.* 2006a); this will not suit the present configuration of the research team. The researchers' epistemological stance is revealed in their previous decision to conduct research using interpretive methods; consequently, these researchers are more likely to select CIS or formal grounded theory than the aggregative and structured thematic synthesis. The application of quality criteria in the selection of primary research in thematic synthesis is likely to be a "sticking point" for the researchers. The actual selection of synthesis method made by these researchers will depend on which criteria in the selection framework are most significant to them. For example, if the costs associated with a particular method will not be covered by funding from a small research grant, the researchers may decide to select a less costly qualitative evidence synthesis method, regardless of the epistemological fit or the expected outcomes of the method.

About this book

I have introduced qualitative evidence synthesis and provided a general overview of the various synthesis methods in this chapter. I have not described any of the synthesis methods in detail. However, the authors of this book will present worked examples of four qualitative evidence synthesis methods in much greater depth. Britten and Pope have written a chapter about meta-ethnography. Flemming has written a chapter on CIS and Crandell, Voils, and Sandelowski have authored a chapter on Bayesian synthesis. Wong describes realist synthesis and Pearson and Hannes discuss meta-aggregation. Kavanagh, Thomas, and Harden provide a chapter about mixed methods. The concluding chapter of the book is written by Manning; he discusses the continuing issues and the future directions in the field of qualitative evidence synthesis. This remarkable team of authors is known worldwide for their expertise and thoughtful critiques of qualitative evidence synthesis. Together they present one of the most practical guides to qualitative evidence

Table 1.1 Synthesis terms introduced in this chapter

Term	Definition
Aggregative method	Qualitative evidence synthesis methods that combine and amalgamate the research findings of primary research in order to produce a summary or overall description of the phenomenon under study. Concepts must be identified in advance. There is no interpretation of how the context of the primary research influences the findings. Requires that the primary research studies are basically comparable in terms of research method and research question. (Noblit & Hare 1998; Estabrooks *et al.* 1994)
Bayesian meta-analysis	The application and extension of traditional Bayesian approaches in meta-analysis. Qualitative evidence is used to determine the variables to be considered in a meta-analysis and their effect sizes. Quantitative evidence constitutes the data in Bayesian meta-analysis. (Roberts *et al.* 2002)
Bayesian synthesis	An adaptation of Bayesian meta-analysis that allows for the equal contribution of both qualitative and quantitative data in the synthesis of research evidence. (Voils *et al.* 2009)
Content analysis	Use of content data analysis strategies to determine frequency of categories of data within a body of primary research. Based on the a priori identification of specific categories of data to ensure consistency between data coders. (Cavanagh 1997; Nandy & Sarvela 1997)
Case survey	A highly structured approach entailing the systematic coding of data from a number of qualitative cases and applying statistical data analysis techniques. (Yin 2003; Yin & Heald 1975)
Critical interpretive synthesis	An adaptation of meta-ethnography, as well as grounded theory, in the synthesis of both qualitative and quantitative evidence. Entails a highly iterative approach to refining the research question and obtaining the primary research sample, as well as data analysis. Also applies a method of assessing quality of primary research studies according to their contribution to theory development rather than methodological attributes. (Dixon-Woods *et al.* 2006a, b)
Ecological triangulation	Also called "ecological sentence synthesis." Applies the concept of triangulation, in which phenomena are studied from a variety of lenses and perspectives. Focuses on theory, method, interventions, populations, environments, and outcomes, as well as relationships among the foci. (Banning 2003; Dixon-Krausse 2006)

(Continued)

Table 1.1   (Continued)

Term	Definition
Formal grounded theory	Adoption of the procedures of grounded theory to synthesize qualitative evidence in grounded theory primary research reports to generate theory about the phenomenon under study. Incorporates the hallmarks of grounded theory, such as theoretical sampling and constant comparative analysis. (Kearney, 1988, 2001)
Framework synthesis	Based on framework analysis previously developed by Pope, Ziebland, and Mays (2000). A deductive approach that uses an a priori "framework," that has been derived from the researchers' discussions and a preliminary literature review, to synthesize the qualitative research findings. Produces a map of each key dimension identified in the synthesis and the nature of their influence and association with other dimensions. (Brunton *et al.* 2006)
Interpretive method	Entails inductive and interpretive processes. Primary purpose is to generate a higher order understanding of the phenomenon under study by generating a theory, model, or concept that overarches the primary research findings represented in the synthesis. (Dixon-Woods *et al.* 2006b)
Meta-analysis	Aggregation of quantitative research findings using pre-selected inclusion and exclusion criteria. Entails an estimation of overall effect-size of the primary research derived from the effect sizes of each individual study. (Glass *et al.* 1981)
Meta-ethnography	An approach that (1) translates the findings of different primary research studies into each other to generate overarching themes, concepts, or metaphors (reciprocal translational analysis); (2) identifies and explains contradictions and differences that exist between the various studies (refutational synthesis); and (3) develops a picture of the whole phenomenon under study from studies of its parts (line-of-argument synthesis). (Noblit & Hare 1988)
Meta-narrative	An exploration of ways of understanding a particular phenomenon across disciplines and research traditions that results in the identification of significant storylines, or meta-narratives, that exist within the field of study. A central focus is explaining differences and contradictions within the body of evidence. (Greenhalgh *et al.* 2005)

(Continued)

Table 1.1   (Continued)

Term	Definition
Meta-study	A multifaceted approach to qualitative evidence synthesis that entails three concurrent components of analysis (i.e., meta-data-analysis, meta-method, and meta-theory), followed by synthesis. The goal of meta-study is to generate new insights or directions in the field of study. It accounts for historical and sociocultural factors that shape the research findings, methods, and theories in a body of primary research. (Paterson *et al.* 2001; Watkins *et al.* 2010)
Meta-summary	An aggregative approach using quantitative techniques to calculate frequency and effect sizes of qualitative data. Primary research findings are summarized to produce a map of the findings according to their frequency and validity. Qualitative meta-summaries can occur as an end to themselves or can form the basis for further synthesis. (Sandelowski & Barroso 2007; Martsolf *et al.* 2010)
Narrative summary	A general description of the findings of selected primary research studies that summarizes the major themes and provides an overview of study findings and relevant issues. Often considered the same as a literature review. (Evans & Kowanko 2000; Sleutel 2000)
Narrative synthesis	Approach that has three steps: developing a preliminary synthesis of the primary research, exploring and describing relationships between the data, and appraising the synthesis product in order to explain and identify moderators for the relationships between data. Entails a well-defined and systematic analytical process. (Spencer *et al.* 2003; Vallido *et al.* 2010)
Systematic review	Entails a comprehensive search for relevant studies on a specific topic and a critical appraisal of the selected research based on pre-determined explicit criteria. Also uses statistical procedures to correct for bias in studies arising most often from sampling error or measurement error. (Tranfield 2006; Booth 2001)
Thematic analysis	The systematic identification of significant, reoccurring, or most common themes in the body of primary research and summarizing these under thematic headings. Can be quantitative (i.e., as in content analysis, themes can be counted and tabulated) but in general is qualitative. (Dixon-Woods *et al.* 2006b; Garcia *et al.* 2002)

(Continued)

Table 1.1 (Continued)

Term	Definition
Thematic synthesis	Uses thematic analysis techniques, as well as adaptations from grounded theory and meta-ethnography, to identify themes across primary research studies. Synthesis component entails an iterative process of inductively grouping themes into overarching categories that capture the similarities, differences, and relationships between the themes for the purpose of generating hypotheses about the phenomenon under study. (Thomas *et al.* 2004; Lipworth *et al.* 2010)

synthesis that currently exists. Although the list of methods described in the book is not exhaustive, the content provides an excellent resource for researchers attempting to make sense of the diverse methodological and epistemological perspectives about qualitative evidence synthesis. I celebrate this book as a much needed advance in the field. It is only when experts in the field are willing to share their experience and insights that the conundrums and issues surrounding qualitative evidence synthesis will be effectively addressed.

Conclusions

This chapter has presented an overview of the evolution and current state of qualitative evidence synthesis. It has highlighted the need for qualitative evidence to inform theory, practice, and policy, while at the same time emphasizing the diversity of methodological and epistemological perspectives that exist on qualitative evidence synthesis. The contributions and methods of qualitative evidence synthesis are still evolving; however, honest and thoughtful explorations of these in books such as this will contribute greatly to our understanding of when qualitative evidence synthesis is called for and which methods best suit particular synthesis projects.

References

Banning JH. (2003) Ecological triangulation: An approach for qualitative meta-synthesis (What works for youth with disabilities project: U.S. Department of Education) http://mycahs.colostate.edu/James.H.Banning/PDFs/Ecological%20Triangualtion.pdf [accessed 7 June 2011].

Bélanger E, Rodríguez C. (2008) More than the sum of its parts? A qualitative research synthesis on multi-disciplinary primary care teams. *Journal of Interprofessional Care.* **22**: 587–97.

Booth A. (2001) Cochrane or cock-eyed? How should we conduct systematic reviews of qualitative research? Paper presented at the Qualitative Evidence-Based Practice Conference: Taking a Critical Stance, Coventry University, http://www.leeds.ac.uk/educol/documents/00001724.doc/2001 [accessed 6 June 2011].

Brunton G, Oliver S, Oliver K *et al.* (2006) *Synthesis of research addressing children's, young people's and parents' views of walking and cycling for transport.* EPPI-Centre, Social Science Research Unit, Institute of Education, University of London, London.

Cavanagh S. (1997) Content analysis: Concepts, methods and applications. *Nurse Researcher.* **4**: 5–16.

Dixon-Krausse PM. (2006) Far and creative learning transfer in management development interventions: An ecological triangulation approach to qualitative meta-synthesis. Unpublished doctoral dissertation, Colorado State University.

Dixon-Woods M, Cavers D, Agarwal S *et al.* (2006a) Conducting a critical interpretive synthesis of the literature on access to healthcare by vulnerable groups. *BMC Medical Research Methodology.* **6**: 35.

Dixon-Woods M, Bonas S, Booth A *et al.* (2006b) How can systematic reviews incorporate qualitative research? A critical perspective. *Qualitative Research.* **6**: 27–44.

Estabrooks CA, Field PA, Morse J. (1994) Aggregating qualitative findings: An approach to theory development. *Qualitative Health Research.* **4**: 503–11.

Evans D, Kowanko I. (2000) Literature reviews: Evolution of a research methodology. *Australian Journal of Advanced Nursing.* **18**: 31–36.

Finfgeld DL. (2003) Metasynthesis: The state of the art—So far. *Qualitative Health Research.* **13**: 893–904.

Finlayson KW, Dixon A. (2008) Qualitative meta-synthesis: a guide for the novice. *Nurse Researcher.* **15**: 59–61.

Garcia J, Bricker L, Henderson J *et al.* (2002) Women's views of pregnancy ultrasound: a systematic review. *Birth.* **29**: 225–50.

Garrett Z, Thomas J. (2004) Systematic reviews and their application to research in speech and language therapy: a response to T. R. Pring's 'Ask a silly question: two decades of troublesome trials.' *International Journal of Language & Communication Disorders.* **41**: 95–105.

Glass GV, McGaw B, Smith ML. (1981) *Metaanalysis in Social Research.* Sage, Beverly Hills.

Gough D, Elbourne D. (2002) Systematic research synthesis to inform policy, practice and democratic debate. *Social Policy & Society.* **1**: 225–36.

Greenhalgh T, Robert G, Macfarlane F *et al.* (2005) Storylines of research in diffusion of innovation: a meta-narrative approach to systematic review. *Social Science & Medicine.* **61**: 417–30.

Harden A, Garcia J, Oliver S, Rees R, Shepherd J, Brunton G, Oakley A. (2004) Applying systematic review methods to studies of people's views: an example from public health. *Journal of Epidemiology in Community Health.* **58**: 794–800.

Kearney M. (2001) Enduring love: a grounded formal theory of women's experience of domestic violence. *Research in Nursing & Health.* **24**: 270–82.

Kearney MH. (1988) Ready-to-wear: discovering grounded formal theory. *Research in Nursing & Health.* **21**: 179–86.

Lipworth WL, Davey HM, Carter SM *et al.* (2010) Beliefs and beyond: what can we learn from qualitative studies of lay people's understandings of cancer risk? *Health Expectations.* **13**: 113–24.

Martsolf DS, Draucker CB, Cook CB *et al.* (2010) A meta-summary of qualitative findings about professional services for survivors of sexual violence. *The Qualitative Report.* **15**: 489–506.

McInnes E, Wimpenny P. (2008) Using Qualitative Assessment and Review Instrument software to synthesise studies on older people's views and experiences of falls prevention. *International Journal of Evidence-based Healthcare.* **6**: 337–44.

Nandy BR, Sarvela PD. (1997) Content analysis reexamined: A relevant research method for health education. *American Journal of Health Behavior.* **21**: 222–34.

NHS CRD. (2001) *Undertaking systematic reviews of research on effectiveness: CRD's guidance for those carrying out or commissioning reviews. CRD Report No. 4,* 2nd ed. NHS, York.

Noblit GW, Hare RD. (1988) *Meta-ethnography: Synthesizing Qualitative Studies.* Sage, London.

Paterson B. (2001) The shifting perspectives model of chronic illness. *Journal of Nursing Scholarship.* **33**: 21–26.

Paterson BL, Thorne SE, Jillings C, Canam C. (2001) *Meta-study of Qualitative Health Research: A Practical Guide to Meta-Analysis and Meta-Synthesis.* Sage, Thousand Oaks.

Paterson BL, Dubouloz C-J, Chevrier J, Ashe B, King J, Moldoveanu M. (2009) Conducting qualitative metasynthesis research: insights from a metasynthesis project. *International Journal of Qualitative Methods.* **8**: 22–33.

Pearson A. (2004) Balancing the evidence: incorporating the synthesis of qualitative data into systematic reviews. *JBI Reports.* **2**: 45–64.

Popay J, Roberts H, Sowden A, Petticrew M, Arai L, Rodgers M, Britten N. (2007) *Guidance on the conduct of narrative synthesis in systematic reviews.* http://www lancs ac uk/fass/projects/nssr/2007 [accessed 6 June 2011].

Pope C, Ziebland S, Mays N. (2000) Qualitative research in health care: analysing qualitative data. *British Medical Journal.* **320**: 114–16.

Roberts KA, Dixon-Wood M, Fitzpatrick R *et al.* (2002) Factors affecting the uptake of childhood immunisation: a Bayesian synthesis of qualitative and quantitative evidence. *Lancet.* **360**: 1596–99.

Russell CL. (2005) An overview of the integrative research review. *Progress in Transplantation.* **15**: 8–13.

Sandelowski M, Barroso J. (2007) *Handbook for Synthesizing Qualitative Research.* Springer, New York.

Sandelowski M, Docherty S, Emden C. (1997) Qualitative metasynthesis: issues and techniques. *Research in Nursing & Health.* **20**: 365–71.

Sherwood G. (1999) Meta-synthesis: Merging qualitative studies to develop nursing knowledge. *International Journal of Human Caring.* **3**: 37–42.

Sleutel MR. (2000) Women's experience of abuse: A review of qualitative research. *Issues in Mental Health Nursing.* **19**: 525–39.

Spencer L, Ritchie J, Lewis J, Dillon L. (2003) *Quality in qualitative evaluation: a framework for assessing research evidence.* Government Chief Social Researcher's Office, London.

Thomas J, Harden A. (2008) Methods for the thematic synthesis of qualitative research in systematic reviews. *BMC Medical Research Methodology.* **8**: 45.

Thomas J, Kavanagh J, Tucker H, Burchett H, Tripney J, Oakley A. (2007) Accidental injury, risk-taking behaviour and the social circumstances in which young people live: a systematic review. EPPI-Centre, Social Science Research Unit, Institute of Education, University of London, London.

Thomas J, Sutcliffe K, Harden A *et al.* (2003) *Children and healthy eating: a systematic review of the barriers and facilitators.* EPPI-Centre, Social Science Research Unit, Institute of Education, University of London, London.

Thomas JR, Harden A, Oakley A *et al.* (2004) Integrating qualitative research with trials in systematic reviews: an example from public health. *British Medical Journal.* **328**: 1010–12.

Thorne S, Paterson B. (1998) Shifting images of chronic illness. *Journal of Nursing Scholarship.* **30**: 173–78.

Thorpe G, McArthur M, Richardson B. (2009) Bodily change following faecal stoma formation: qualitative interpretive synthesis. *Journal of Advanced Nursing.* **65**: 1778–89.

Tranfield D. (2006) Using qualitative research synthesis to build an actionable knowledge base. *Management Decisions.* **44**: 213–27.

Vallido T, Wilkes L, Carter B *et al.* (2010) Mothering disrupted by illness: a narrative synthesis of qualitative research. *Journal of Advanced Nursing.* **66**: 1435–45.

Voils CA, Hasselblad V, Crandell JL *et al.* (2009) A Bayesian method for the synthesis of evidence from qualitative and quantitative reports: the example of antiretroviral medication adherence. *Journal of Health Services Research & Policy.* **14**: 226–33.

Walsh D, Downe S. (2005) Meta-synthesis method for qualitative research: a literature review. *Journal of Advanced Nursing.* **50**: 204–11.

Watkins DC, Walker RL, Griffith DM. (2010) A meta-study of black male mental health and well-being. *Journal of Black Psychology.* **36**: 303–30.

Wilson K, Avir Z. (2008) Cancer and disability benefits: a synthesis of qualitative findings on advice and support. *Psychooncology.* **17**: 421–29.

Yager RE. (2006) Factors involved with qualitative syntheses: a new focus for research in science education. *Journal of Research in Science Teaching.* **19**: 337–50.

Yin R. (2003) *Applications of Case Study Research.* Applied Social Research Methods Series Vol **34**. Sage, Thousand Oaks.

Yin RK, Heald KA. (1975) Using the case survey method to analyse policy studies. *Administrative Science Quarterly.* **20**: 371–81.

Zimmer L. (2006) Qualitative meta-synthesis: a question of dialoguing with texts. *Journal of Advanced Nursing.* **53**: 311–18.

Chapter 2 Obstacles to the implementation of evidence-based practice in Belgium: a worked example of meta-aggregation

Karin Hannes, PhD[1] and Alan Pearson, AM[2]

[1]Centre for Methodology of Educational Research, Faculty of Psychology and Education, K.U.Leuven, Belgium and Centre for Evidence-Based Medicine, Belgian Branch of the Cochrane Collaboration, Belgium

[2]Joanna Briggs Institute, Faculty of Health Sciences, University of Adelaide, Australia

Meta-aggregation as a method of synthesis has its roots in the systematic approach outlined by the Cochrane Collaboration. Greatly inspired by the founding fathers of American Pragmatism, it concentrates on the original researchers' processed data and summarizes common and competing findings to produce cross-study generalizations that lead to recommendations for action. Meta-aggregation seeks to generate summaries to determine the value of the findings of individual studies in terms of their practical consequences. The example on barriers towards the implementation of evidence-based practice guides researchers through the main steps of the aggregative approach: the development of a question, the search for evidence, the critical appraisal of original research papers and the aggregation of original findings into categories, and further on into syntheses. We also present the Qualitative Assessment and Review Instrument as an online tool that can support authors in conducting their synthesis.

Introduction

Meta-aggregation is an approach that is increasing in popularity as a method of qualitative synthesis designed to model the Cochrane process of systematic reviews summarizing results of quantitative studies whilst being sensitive to the nature of qualitative research and its traditions (Pearson 2004). Implicit in its development is recognition of the valuable role qualitative research/evidence

---

Synthesizing Qualitative Research: Choosing the Right Approach, First Edition.
Edited by Karin Hannes and Craig Lockwood.
© 2012 John Wiley & Sons, Ltd. Published 2012 by John Wiley & Sons, Ltd.

can play in informing evidence-based healthcare (Joanna Briggs Institute 2009). Flemming (2007) identifies several different approaches that can be used to synthesize qualitative research studies. She distinguishes between interpretive and integrative reviews, the latter aggregative in nature. Estabrooks *et al.* (1994) make a case for undertaking what they call "aggregation" of qualitative studies and define it as ". . . a type of secondary analyses particular to qualitative research" that restricts its focus to studies of similar populations and themes and to studies that adequately report data (the actual words of the participant or the field notes of observers) as well as findings (the results of the researcher's analysis and interpretation). Synthesizing qualitative research findings has the capacity to produce generalizations that not only contribute to theory, but can be of a suggestive, naturalistic, or idiographic nature and may be predictive (Sandelowski *et al.* 1997).

Drawing on the work of Estabrook *et al.* and Sandalowski, Docherty, and Emden, from March 2001, a group of qualitative researchers[1] participated in a participative consensus project that considered how a systematic process of extracting and synthesizing qualitative data can occur to reflect a rigoros process equivalent to the existing processes applied to the results of Randomized Controlled Trials (RCTs) and other quantitative research, but maintaining sensitivity to the contextual nature of qualitative research. The outcome of the project was the development of an aggregative approach to the synthesis of qualitative evidence that:

- emphasized the complexity of interpretive and critical understandings of phenomena;
- recognized the need to ensure that the process is practical and usable;
- balanced utility of the outcomes with the complexity of the material;
- was grounded in pragmatism.

The meta-aggregative approach has been inspired by the work of Charles Sanders Peirce (1877), William James (1909), and John Dewey (1938), who developed respectively extended the philosophy of pragmatism. They subscribed to the theory that knowledge is power and that the value of any thought lies in its practical use and consequences. It is the focus on practical consequences that characterizes meta-aggregation as a synthesis approach.

---

[1] Professor Alan Pearson, The Joanna Briggs Institute, Professor Mary FitzGerald, University of Newcastle; Professor Jane Stein-Parbury, University of Technology, Sydney; Professor Colin Holmes, James Cook University of Northern Queensland; Professor Michael Clinton, Curtin University; Professor Desley Hegney, University of Southern Queensland; Dr Ken Walsh, The University of Adelaide; Dr Karen Francis, Charles Sturt University; Mr Matt Lewis, La Trobe University; and Ms Cathy Ward, La Trobe University.

Central to pragmatism were communities of inquiry or groups of people with a shared interest, problem, or issue trying to resolve doubt through critical reasoning. Decisions were expected to be obtained by gathering and surveying evidence appraised as to its weight and relevancy, and by framing and testing plans of action in their capacity as hypotheses (Dewey 1938). Actions were then expected to be assessed in the light of their practical consequences. In meta-aggregation the actual potential for confrontation between, for example, researchers and practitioners or other target groups, is limited. What acts as the community of inquiry here are the original research manuscripts. Aggregation does not pursue interpretative analysis of the data extracted from original studies. Instead, it concentrates on the original researchers' findings (processed data) and summarizes common and competing findings to produce cross-study generalizations that lead to recommendations for action. It aims to balance the complexity of the research material from original qualitative papers with the utility of the outcomes for practitioners and policymakers. It is in the theoretical exercise of categorizing findings to arrive at a set of meaningful recommendations that theory and practice actually meet.

A worked example

This worked example originates from a personal interest in aspects influencing the implementation of evidence-based practice (EBP). The general idea of evidence-based practice is to use insights from recent and high quality scientific studies to support clinical decision-making has been welcomed by many different disciplines in healthcare. However, a number of barriers have hampered its implementation in daily care. Some of the obstacles seem to be universal and have been reported by authors from different countries, such as time constraints and inadequate facilities, including limited access to information resources (Parrilla-Castellar *et al.* 2008; Sharek *et al.* 2008; Zaidi *et al.*; 2007; Rabe *et al.* 2007; Khoja & Al-Ansary 2007; Adib-Hajbaghery 2007; Grimmer-Somers *et al.* 2007). Other obstacles appear to be more specific and relate to the unique identity of certain disciplines in healthcare, such as the lack of authority and cooperation from physicians mentioned by nurses (Hannes *et al.* 2007; Chau *et al.* 2008), financial concerns stated by physicians (Hannes *et al.* 2005), and the difficulties in defining clear outcome measures in the field of physiotherapy and psychiatry (Swinkels *et al.* 2002; Grimmer-Somers 2007; Hannes *et al.* 2009a; Hannes *et al.* 2009b). Reviews summarizing insights from qualitative, empirical studies on barriers to EBP are absent. The meta-aggregation presented sets out to begin to fill this gap. The overall aim of this qualitative evidence synthesis was to examine the commonalities in the obstacles experienced by a broad range of healthcare practitioners. A context-specific synthesis, focusing on the Belgian healthcare system, was opted for. This choice facilitates the development of recommendations for Belgian practitioners and policymakers, which is one of the core goals of a meta-aggregative approach.

The process of meta-aggregation

The process used drew on the methods of QARI: the Qualitative Assessment and Review Instrument (Joanna Briggs Institute 2003). This process (summarized in Figure 2.1) includes the development of a review question; the conduct of a comprehensive search; the critical appraisal of studies selected for retrieval; extraction of findings; and the meta-aggregation of findings. As Figure 2.1 shows, studies using different methodologies can be included in one review. When findings are extracted, they are aggregated into a single set of categories which are then further aggregated to generate synthesized findings.

The QARI software guides meta-aggregation as part of a systematic review. QARI was designed as a web-based application and developed to provide a structured process for systematically reviewing qualitative evidence and arriving at an evidence synthesis. It incorporates a critical appraisal instrument; data extraction forms; a data synthesis function; and a reporting function. It mirrors the process taken for systematic reviews of quantitative research. The QARI software allows for transparency and leaves an audit trail for others to follow and/or replicate.

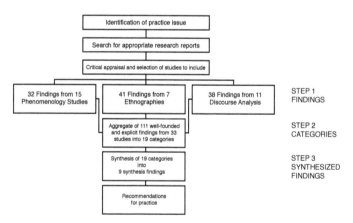

Figure 2.1   Steps in the systematic review and meta-aggregation of qualitative studies. Reproduced with permission from the Joanna Briggs Institute, Reviewers' Manual, 2008.

Question development

To be able to focus our meta-aggregation a scoping review was carried out to identify the type of reviews already published. All of the published qualitative evidence syntheses brought together the findings on one particular target group and aimed to give a broader international perspective. No examples of qualitative evidence syntheses were found that particularly searched for and focused on country-specific issues including, for example, perspectives from different target groups living or working in the same environment and between the boundaries of a socio-cultural, economic, and local political system. Given the context-specific nature of qualitative research we opted for a qualitative evidence synthesis based on the findings of scientific studies addressing the barriers to the implementation of EBP of Belgian healthcare practitioners only. Meta-aggregation was an obvious choice of method for this research project. More than other approaches it produces synthesized statements that allow for the development of recommendations for policy and practice, which was one of the goals of the project. The PICo mnemonic was used to frame our research question.

- *Population*: healthcare practitioners
- *Phenomena of Interest*: obstacles towards the implementation of evidence-based practice
- *Context*: Belgian healthcare system
- *Outcome*: experiences and perceptions

The following questions needed to be answered by the synthesis: What are the obstacles towards implementing EBP experienced or perceived by healthcare practitioners working in the Belgian healthcare system? Which obstacles cut across the different disciplines and what advice can be given to practice and policy to enable them to bridge these obstacles?

Search strategy and inclusion criteria

The components of the research question assisted us in formulating our inclusion criteria for the review. To be considered for the meta-aggregation original research reports were subjected to the following evaluation:

- *Study type*: Qualitative, empirical research papers. Opinion pieces and descriptive articles were excluded.
- *Study participants*: All types of healthcare practitioners, e.g. physicians, dentists, nurses, physiotherapists, psychologists.
- *Topic of interest*: Obstacles to the implementation of EBP.
- *Context*: The Belgian healthcare system.
- *Outcome of interest*: Experiences and/or perceptions from participants.

The search strategy developed for this evidence synthesis aimed at finding both published and unpublished studies. We searched Medline, CINAHL, Psychinfo, Embase, Social Sciences abstracts, and ERIC to retrieve relevant studies (1990–May 2008). We used keywords associated with the broad topic of "Evidence-Based Practice (Medical Subject Heading (MeSH) term)", including Evidence-Based Dentistry, Nursing, and Medicine. Additional keywords such as evidence-based were combined with the geographical notion "Belgian," "Flemish/Flanders", or "Walloon." Where possible we used a methodological filter for qualitative research. We further searched the "Federal research actions" database from the Belgian governmental department of science and consulted Belgian experts in qualitative research methods and/or evidence-based practice to check on any other published material that could be of use for the synthesis.

Description of the included studies
Eight studies met our inclusion criteria: a series of five papers written by the lead author (Hannes *et al.* 2005 (GPs), Hannes *et al.* 2007 (nurses), Hannes *et al.* 2008b (dentists), Hannes *et al.* 2008a (psychiatrists), Hannes *et al.* 2009a (physiotherapists), and three additional reports retrieved via local literature and contacts. The five studies of Hannes and colleagues were explorative and described the experiences of 245 Belgian (Dutch speaking) healthcare practitioners: 31 general practitioners, 53 nurses, 43 physiotherapists, and 39 psychiatrists. Four studies used the technique of focus groups to collect data and comparative analysis, guided by a grounded theory approach, to analyze the set of data. For the study on dentists a thematic analysis was used. Van Driel *et al.* (2003) interviewed 17 individual general practitioners. They addressed barriers to EBP, particularly clinical guidelines. The study was explorative and geographically limited to East, West, and Zeeuws-Flanders. Insights generated in the Netherlands (Zeeuws-Flanders) could not be separated from those identified in Belgium. We chose to include this study. A thematic analysis was used for analysis purposes. Autrique *et al.* (2007) interviewed 60 persons: 11 psychologists, 10 heads of psychiatric departments, 8 directors, 5 clinical-therapeutical coordinators, and several psychiatrists. Twenty-eight were working in Walloon healthcare institutes and 32 were related to Flemish institutes. All of them worked with addicts. Data analysis was based on the case-oriented quantification approach from Kuckartz (1998). A report and article were published, based on the same original data. We included findings from the report, since it was the most comprehensive and detailed from both options. Heymans *et al.* (2006) reported on data from 12 focus groups, in which 93 (45 Walloon and 48 Flemish) general practitioners participated. A deductive approach

was used to analyse data, starting from a matrix with predefined categories of obstacles retrieved from a literature search. New findings were added to the matrix.

Quality assessment

Critical appraisal of qualitative studies is a particularly contested issue in relation to qualitative evidence synthesis. Some argue that criteria are best regarded as guides to good practice, rather than as rigid requirements in appraising papers (Spencer *et al.* 2003). Some even call for an end to "criteriology," arguing that it stifles the interpretative and creative aspects of qualitative research (Sandelowski & Barroso 2003). Reviewers who support the meta-aggregative approach consider a transparent approach to appraising qualitative research – sensitive to the nature of qualitative research and its basis in subjectivity – central to its ongoing credibility, transferability, and theoretical potential (Pearson, 2004). Therefore, a critical appraisal instrument is integrated into the QARI software to facilitate this process. This instrument assesses congruity between the philosophical/theoretical position adopted in the study, study methodology, study methods and the research question, the representation of the data, and the interpretation of the findings. It further evaluates the degree to which the values, beliefs, and potential influences of the researcher on the project are made explicit and the relationship between what the participants are reported to have said/done and the conclusions drawn in analysis. Ethics are also considered. The JBI appraisal instrument provides a coherent set of appraisal criteria. Two independent reviewers are required to complete this appraisal process. Any conflicts can be solved by involving a third reviewer.

The worked example presented did not include a systematic assessment of quality. Reasons for this are the limited amount of studies found and the fact that the majority of these studies were written by the lead reviewer, who would also be one of the appraisers. An overall judgment approach was used instead. This approach has been proved to deliver more or less the same outcome as a checklist approach (Dixon-Woods 2007). However, it tends to be less explicit about potential reasons for exclusion. Therefore, an evaluation based on the JBI-critical appraisal instrument incorporated in the QARI software is recommended for other review teams opting for a meta-aggregative approach to synthesis.

Qualitative data analysis

The process of evidence synthesis involved the extraction of the details (methods, setting, type of participants etc.) from each original study included and the aggregation of original findings into categories and further on into

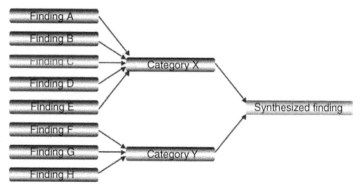

Figure 2.2 Display of end result in QARI software.

syntheses. The typical outcome produced by following the structure outlined in the QARI software is presented in Figure 2.2 above.

One reviewer extracted and analyzed the findings. The use of two independent data-extractors is not required within the meta-aggregative approach. However, when it comes to moving from original findings to categories, synthesized findings, and recommendations the benefit of using more than one reviewer lies in the multiple perspectives that colleagues can bring to the scene, which helps deepening understanding. To improve the trustworthiness of the synthesis the authors of original studies other than those produced by the lead reviewer were contacted to establish their response to our interpretation of the papers. An email request to comment on the draft of the synthesis was sent out. All lead authors responded with constructive comments to enhance the synthesis. Involving the authors of the included studies has been a very positive experience. However, each suggestion made needs to be traced back to the original dataset to check whether it is indeed grounded in the data, before it can be added to the synthesis. This has been a time-consuming process.

Step 1: Extracting the findings
The first step in this process involves reviewers extracting all of the findings from each of the included papers. A finding is defined as a theme, category, or metaphor reported by authors of original papers. These are generally supported with illustrations from participants' voices (interview or observation excerpts, citations, etc.) that demonstrate the origins of the findings. The general idea of meta-aggregation is to stay as close as possible to the themes (usually underlined or in bold) listed by the original authors and prevent interpretation occurring in this phase of the review. Most studies in our synthesis presented coherent themes, such as "characteristics of evidence," "characteristics of doctors,"

"colleagues," "government," and/or "the healthcare system." Other themes presented included "characteristics of patients and family," "the media," "commercial organizations," "management," "characteristics of the discipline," "the personal characteristics of the practitioner," "attitudes," "guidelines," "the environment," or "external factors." We also found themes related to "the applicability of evidence" and to "clinical experience (as opposed to scientific research)." As much as we wanted to stay close to the original categories used in defining what the findings were, many did not really succeed in pinning down the real obstacles. Names used to categorize original findings were generally broad in scope and most of these themes captured several meaningful ideas. We expected that it would result in findings that would need a broad range of citations as a back-up to be able to capture the whole meaning. Therefore, it was decided to screen each theme mentioned in the original papers for emerging obstacles. These obstacles were labeled as 'findings' for the synthesis. The statements made by the original authors in their papers were particularly helpful in doing this. Whenever a citation was available to back-up the findings retrieved from the original report we used it to illustrate or support our finding. Interview excerpts were actively searched for. Levels of credibility were then assigned to the findings based on whether or not they were sufficiently grounded in the data. QARI software allows reviewers to use three "levels of evidence" for the findings and later the conclusions deriving from the synthesis: "unequivocal," "credible," and "unsupported" (Pearson *et al.* 2004). A different label was assigned to findings with citations that supported them beyond reasonable doubt (unequivocal) or citations that were open to challenge and interpretation (credible). The meta-aggregative approach does not outline whether or not unsupported statements, that is findings without supporting citations, should be taken along in reviews other than those submitted to their institutional database (these authors do not report on unsupported findings). It was our decision to include them, given the fact that many authors face word restrictions by journal editors. However, they should be read and interpreted with caution. It was decided to report them alongside the findings in our report, mainly because it enables readers to evaluate the trustworthiness of the findings (Figure 2.3). We further decided to cluster findings that were similar for different disciplines, indicating for which professional groups a finding would hold true. This also was a personal choice of the reviewers. Figure 2.3 displays one of the four syntheses derived and provides more detailed information about how the results from step 1 might be reported.

Other acceptable ways of reporting step 1 are to count the number of findings that can be assigned to a certain category, display the number in the figure instead of its content, and list the original findings in an annex. This

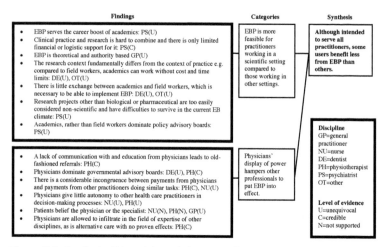

Figure 2.3   Synthesis: Although intended to serve all practitioners, some users benefit less from EBP than others. Reproduced from Hannes K, Goedhuys J & Aertgeerts B. Obstacles to implementing Evidence-Based Practice in Belgium: a context-specific qualitative evidence synthesis including findings from different health care disciplines. *Acta Clinica Belgica* (in press), with permission from Acta Clinica Belgica.

strategy has recently been used in a review on "The psychosocial spiritual experience of elderly individuals recovering from stroke" (Lamb *et al.* 2008). Figure 2.4 displays one of the four syntheses as an example.

Step 2: Categorizing findings
The second step in meta-aggregation involves an evaluation of the similarity in meaning of the findings that cut across the different original papers. To

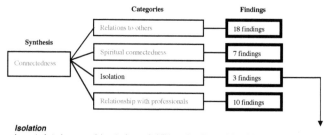

Figure 2.4   Connectedness. Reproduced from Hannes K, Goedhuys J & Aertgeerts B. Obstacles to implementing Evidence-Based Practice in Belgium: a context-specific qualitative evidence synthesis including findings from different health care disciplines. *Acta Clinica Belgica* (in press), with permission from Acta Clinica Belgica.

prevent us from ending up with categories that were too general to reveal useful information in the first place we decided on full sentences to present our categories. Instead of using broad titles such as "obstacles related to medical doctors" or "attitudes" we translated these into "medical doctors' display of power hampers practitioners to put EBP in practice" and "attitudes of practitioners hinder the implementation of EBP."

The meta-aggregation revealed 9 categories derived from 147 findings:

- *Category 1: Evidence is hard to implement.*
This category reports on obstacles related to the accessibility of information, the limited applicability of research results, and the suboptimal reporting of scientific reports not revealing information that is relevant for practitioners.
- *Category 2: Decision making processes are influenced by patient variables.*
This category covers for issues such as (emancipated) patients' expectations and uniqueness, influences of the media, and the tendency to adapt to the patients' wishes.
- *Category 3: Decision-making processes are influenced by practitioner variables.*
Issues such as practitioner habits, skills, knowledge of previous events, threats to therapeutic freedom, and so on dominate this category.
- *Category 4: Commercial/financial interests affect EBP.*
The main focus within this category is the potential influence of drug and other companies on the outcome of scientific studies and the fact that academic careers are intertwined with industrial partnership. It also addresses the economic interests of government, managers in institutes, and practitioners themselves.
- *Category 5: Governmental regulations influence the process of implementation.*
This category reports on the top-down approach and contra-productivity of governmental decisions, its lack of control and incentives, as well as the fact that the current reimbursement system is outdated for many topics.
- *Category 6: EBP is more feasible for practitioners working in a scientific setting compared to those working in other settings.*
Apart from cost and time limit issues for practitioners in the field, this category also focuses on the strong representation of academics in advisory boards, and the lack of support to combine both practice and research.
- *Category 7: Physicians' display of power hampers other professionals to put evidence-based practice into effect.*
Concepts such as power, authority, hierarchy, and dominance of physicians as compared to allied health professionals are the main focus of this category. It addresses incongruence in payments, old fashioned referrals practitioners are bound to, and infiltration of physicians in other fields of healthcare.

- *Category 8: A lack of knowledge and skills hinders the implementation of evidence-based practice.*
  In this category gaps in medical curricula, knowledge gaps between younger and older colleagues, lack of expertise of teachers and supervisors, difficulties of having to read foreign languages, and the newness of the concept of EBP are addressed.
- *Category 9: Attitudes of healthcare practitioners hinder the implementation of EBP.*
  This category reveals the lack of motivation or willingness to act in an evidence-based manner and the resistance towards the whole evidence-based movement, which is stated to be partially linked to personalities of practitioners and partly to certain disciplines in healthcare.

In contrast with the process of identifying the findings, the process of deciding on the categories did involve interpretation. In starting to think about grouping findings according to similarity in meaning and naming them accordingly it was noticed that discussion between researchers helps to better shape the categories, for example category 4 and 5 were initially bundled in one category on economic interests affecting EBP. It was not until the discussion phase that we became aware of a potential bias in interpretation. We had focused on the economic interests of government without noticing that, for example, reimbursement issues could also have been caused by lack of knowledge or structural barriers in keeping the healthcare system regulations up to date. These aspects were filtered out and an extra category "governmental regulations" was created. These categories were then brought together in a synthesis. The final synthesis was formulated more broadly than "economics," focusing on "aspects other than quality of care steering the EBP agenda," as is outlined in Figure 2.5.

Category 1 was rather broad in scope and included so many findings that we decided to develop subcategories with the findings in the report. QARI software, however, does not allow reviewers to use such subcategories. It was a personal choice of the reviewers to do so (Figure 2.6).

Step 3: Synthesizing categories
The reviewer needs to review the full list of categories developed and identify sufficient similarity in meaning to generate a comprehensive set of synthesized findings. The nine categories in this worked example were summarized in order to produce four syntheses that could be used as a basis to inform evidence-based practice and policy. In meta-aggregation a synthesized finding is defined as an overarching description of a group of categorized findings that allow for the generation of recommendations for practice. The synthesized statements should help us to consider possible lines of action and will make our responses more precise. Meta-aggregation prefers a declam-

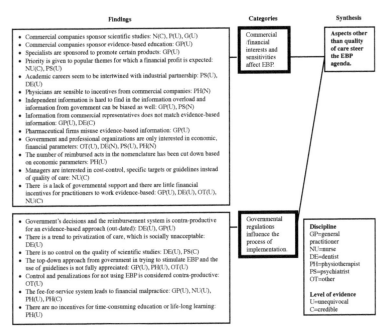

Figure 2.5 Synthesis: Aspects other than quality of care steer the EBP agenda. Reproduced from Hannes K, Goedhuys J & Aertgeerts B. Obstacles to implementing Evidence-Based Practice in Belgium: a context-specific qualitative evidence synthesis including findings from different health care disciplines. *Acta Clinica Belgica* (in press), with permission from Acta Clinica Belgica.

atory form of formulating the synthesis that emphasizes the probability of the claim, as is demonstrated in the formulation of the four syntheses derived from the worked example below:

- *Synthesis 1*: Evidence might have a limited role in decision-making processes in daily practice, if the importance of the scientific component in the decision making process is not stressed (categories 1, 2, and 3).
- *Synthesis 2*: Aspects other than quality of care will steer the EBP agenda, if governmental regulations and economic interests do not entirely focus on the delivery of the best possible care (categories 4 and 5).
- *Synthesis 3*: Although EBP is intended to serve all practitioners, some healthcare providers will benefit less from EBP than others if inequity issues between practitioners and support for field workers are not considered (categories 6 and 7).
- *Synthesis 4*: A lack of competences will hinder the implementation of EBP, if gaps in knowledge and skills are not being filled and efforts to change contra-productive attitudes are not undertaken (categories 8 and 9).

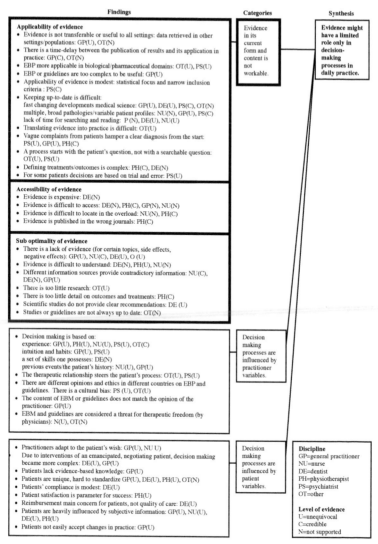

Figure 2.6 Synthesis: Evidence might have a limited role in decision-making processes in daily practice. Reproduced from Hannes K, Goedhuys J & Aertgeerts B. Obstacles to implementing Evidence-Based Practice in Belgium: a context-specific qualitative evidence synthesis including findings from different health care disciplines. *Acta Clinica Belgica* (in press), with permission from Acta Clinica Belgica.

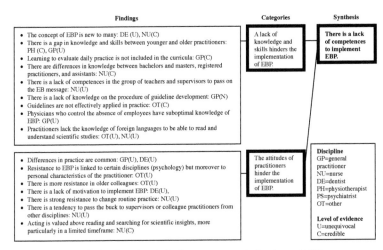

Figure 2.7 Synthesis: There is a lack of competences to implement EBP.

It was noticed that in this phase theoretical frameworks and reviewers' schools of thought were at play. The researchers had a heated discussion on whether or not attitudes of practitioners should be considered under the main heading "lack of competences" or elsewhere. Those with an educational background were highly in favor of bringing knowledge, skills, and attitudes together. The concept of competences in pedagogy is defined as the compilation of knowledge, skills, and attitudes that steer someone's professional behavior and acting. Those with a more clinical background argued that a separate category of "attitudes" could cover additional ideas broader than competences, such as the concern that it is something for academics rather than practitioners working in the field. In moving from categories to syntheses the different perspectives from co-reviewers enabled the team to better motivate the final choices made and reflect on the influence their background was bringing to the scene (Figure 2.7).

All four syntheses derived via this worked example have been displayed within step one, two, and three. However, to be workable the synthesized statements displayed in Figures 2.3 and 2.5 to 2.7 had to be reformulated into clear lines of action (step 3). Meta-aggregation specifically stresses the fact that we cannot exclude acts of choice on what particular direction to take with the outcome of a synthesis from the responsibility of the reviewer. It is particularly in this phase that there will always be some degree of interpretation involved. The declamatory form of formulating the synthesis helped the authors in formulating suggestions to practitioners and policy makers on how to move forward with the results of the review. What adds to the robustness of the approach is that these cues to action can always be traced back to the original data in the supporting software QARI.

Step 4: Recommendations and advice

Implications for practice and policy

- Consider educating patients and exploring potential information channels that influence patients' opinions to create space for well-informed decisions (synthesis 1).
- Provide easy and free access to well-structured, compact, and relevant information targeted to a particular discipline and consider helpdesks. Screen information, control its quality, and translate it to the field (synthesis 1).
- Consider updating the Belgian nomenclature and reimbursement system to bring it in line with the latest evidence (synthesis 2).
- Consider incentives for those practitioners who are engaging themselves in the implementation of EBP in daily practice, to keep them motivated and to prevent creation of a negative spiral in which practitioners tend to believe that efforts to improve practice automatically lead to a loss of income (synthesis 2).
- Enhance communication and cooperation between physicians and other partners in healthcare, via their professional groups and journals (synthesis 3).
- Consider programs tailored to the needs of specific disciplines and stimulate multidisciplinary education to create mutual understanding across disciplines (synthesis 3, 4).
- Consider direct access to allied health services to increase autonomy (synthesis 3).
- Integrate EBP in the basic curricula (synthesis 4).

Implications for future research

- Research projects based on observation techniques would create an opportunity to explore in more detail what the interfering factors in decision-making processes are (synthesis 1).
- Consider a shift from the question of what the barriers are to the question of how evidence contributes to a particular clinical decision and in what circumstances it fails to do so (synthesis 1).
- Provide financial incentives for research that is not picked up by pharmacy. This implies openness for designs that do not directly fit the scope of, for example, RCTs as well as preserving budgets for strategic domains in all disciplines in healthcare and for different schools of thought within these disciplines (synthesis 2).
- Consider previous research on change strategies to motivate practitioners and break down the resistance towards EBP in the field (synthesis 4).

Discussion

Although the methodology of meta-aggregation has been well-described in user guides and well-supported through the software QARI, some choices had to be made that might have impacted on the results of the synthesis. Firstly, we chose to synthesize findings from accepted or published papers only. By doing so, we enabled the readers to evaluate the trustworthiness of the synthesis. The references to the original papers or articles enable the reader to look back at the basic findings. However, we cannot guarantee that all relevant insights were included in the study. Unlike some other researchers who have conducted meta-aggregations (Briggs & Fleming 2007) we chose to report all study findings, including those that were not supported with quotes from the original studies. We felt that one of the major reasons for this lack of support might be the limited word space in the journals to which the studies were submitted. We double checked all "unsupported" statements in our own studies and found evidence for all of them in the original dataset. It is advisable for other reviewers who choose to exclude non-supported statements to contact authors from original papers when evidence appears to be missing. Secondly, the evidence synthesis includes studies which differ in their study question. All studies investigated barriers, however some mentioned barriers to EBP whilst pursuing other remits. In order not to exclude potentially useful findings, we included studies that identified barriers, although they were not necessarily a primary focus of the research (Heymans *et al.* 2006; Autrique *et al.* 2007; Van Driel *et al.* 2003). The meta-aggregation presented does not replace the need for original research. However, with its aim to arrive at a set of suggestions to inform practice and policy it allows for greater control over the problematic situations practitioners and policy-makers are confronted with in the field of healthcare. It has certainly proved to be a very useful approach to address our research question.

Acknowledgements

Thanks to Jo Goedhuys and Bert Aertgeerts for assisting in developing the research objectives and to Willy Peetermans for reflecting on the categorization and final syntheses. A special thanks to the QARI Development Group, who has made a major contribution in developing study guides on the meta-aggregative approach.

References

Adib-Hajbaghery M. (2007) 'Factors facilitating and inhibiting evidence-based nursing in Iran'. *J Adv Nurs*. Jun; **58**(6): 566–75.

Autrique M, Vanderplasschen W, Thierry HP, Broekaert E, Sabbe B. (2007) *Evidence-Based werken in de verslavingszorg: een stand van zaken*. Academia Press, Gent: 113–156.

Briggs M, Flemming K. (2007) Living with leg ulceration: a synthesis of qualitative research. *J Adv Nurs*. Aug; **59**(4): 319–28. Epub 2007 Jul 2.

Chau JP, Lopez V, Thompson DR. (2008) A survey of Hong Kong nurses' perceptions of barriers to and facilitators of research utilization. *Res Nurs Health*. Jun 3.

Dewey J. (1938) *Logic: The Theory of Inquiry*. New York: Holt and Company.

Dixon-Woods M, Sutton A, Shaw R, Miller T, Smith J, Young B, Bonas S, Booth A, Jones D. (2007) Appraising qualitative research for inclusion in systematic reviews: a quantitative and qualitative comparison of three methods. *J Health Serv Res Policy*. **12**(1): 42–7.

Estabrooks, C.C., Field, P.A., Morse, J.M. (1994) Aggregating qualitative findings: An approach to theory development. *Qualitative Health Research*. **4**: 503–511.

Flemming K. (2007) The synthesis of qualitative research and evidence-based nursing. *Evid Based Nurs*. **10**(3): 68–71.

Grimmer-Somers K, Lekkas P, Nyland L, Young A, Kumar S. (2007) Perspectives on research evidence and clinical practice: a survey of Australian physiotherapists. *Physiother Res Int*. **12**(3): 147–61.

Hannes K, Leys M, Buntinx F, Vermeire E, Aertgeerts B, Depoorter AM. (2005) Implementing evidence-based medicine in general practice: a focus group based study. *BMC-Family Practice*. **6**(37): 1–13.

Hannes K, Vandersmissen J, De Blaeser L, Goedhuys J, Peeters G, Schepers R, Aertgeerts B. (2007) Barriers to evidence-based nursing: a focus group study. *Journal of Advanced Nursing*. **60**(2): 162–71.

Hannes K, Pieters G, Simons W, Herman G, Aertgeerts B. (2008a) Preliminaire resultaten van een focusgroepen onderzoek over hinderpalen in de implementatie van Evidence-Based Praktijkvoering in Vlaanderen: Zijn psychiaters anders dan andere hulpverleners? *Tijdschrift voor psychiatrie*. **50**(6): 345–52.

Hannes K, Norré D, Goedhuys J, Naert I, Aertgeerts B. (2008b) Barriers to the implementation of evidence-based dentistry: a focus group based study. *Journal of Dental Education*. **72**(6): 736–44.

Hannes K, Staes F, Vangesselen S, Goedhuys J, Aertgeerts B. (2009a) Implementing evidence-based physiotherapy: a focus group based study. *Physiotherapy Theory and Practice*. **25**(7): 476–88.

Hannes K, Pieters G, Goedhuys J, Aertgeerts B. (2009b) Exploring barriers to the implementation of evidence-based practice in psychiatry to inform health policy: a focus group based study. *Community Ment Health J*. Nov 4.

Heymans I, Van Linden A, Mambourg F, Leys M. (2006) Feedback: onderzoek naar de impact en barrières bij implementatie – Onderzoeksrapport: deel II. *Federal Knowledge Centre for Health Care reports* vol. 32A, 49–61.

Joanna Briggs, Institute., (2003) JBI-Meta Analysis of Statistics Assessment and Review Instrument: SUMARI package Validity Checklist. JBI, Adelaide.

Joanna Briggs, Institute., (2007) The Joanna Briggs Institute system for the unified management, assessment and review of information. User Guide Version 4.0.

James W. (1909) *The Meaning of Truth*. Longman Green and Co, New York, 1909.

Khoja TA, Al-Ansary LA. (2007) Attitudes to evidence-based medicine of primary care physicians in Asir region, Saudi Arabia. *East Mediterr Health J.* **13**(2): 408–19.

Kuckartz U. WinMax (1998) *Scientific Text Analysis for the Social Sciences – A User Guide.* BSS, Berlin.

Lamb, M., D. Buchanan, *et al.* (2008). The psychosocial spiritual experience of elderly individuals recovering from stroke: a systematic review. *International Journal of Evidence-Based Health Care* **6**(2): 173–205.

Parrilla-Castellar ER, Almeyda R, Nogales E, Vélez M, Ramos M, Rivera JE, Dá Vila B, Torres V, Capriles J, Adamsons K. (2008) Evidence-based medicine as a tool for clinical decision-making in Puerto Rico. *P R Health Sci J.* **27**(2): 135–40.

Pearson A. (2004) Balancing the evidence: Incorporating the synthesis of qualitative data into systematic reviews. *JBI Reports.* **2**: 45–64.

Peirce CS. (1877) The fixation of belief. *Popular Science Monthly,* **12** November, P 1–15.

Rabe P, Holmén A, Sjögren P. (2007) Attitudes, awareness and perceptions on evidence based dentistry and scientific publications among dental professionals in the county of Halland, Sweden: a questionnaire survey. *Swed Dent J.* **31**(3): 113–20.

Sandelowski, M. Docherty, S. and Embden, C. (1997). Focus on kwalitatieve methods. Qualitative meta-synthesis: Issues and techniques. *Research and Nursing in Health.* **20**(4): 365–71.

Sandelowski M & Barroso J. (2003) Toward a meta-synthesis of qualitative findings on motherhood in HIV-positive women. *Research Nursing and Health.* **26**: 153–170.

Sharek PJ, Mullican C, Lavanderos A, Palmer C, Snow V, Kmetik K, Antman M, Knutson D, Dembry LM. (2007) Best practice implementation: lessons learned from 20 partnerships. *Jt Comm J Qual Patient Saf.* **33**(12 Suppl): 16–26.

Spencer L, Ritchie J, Lewis J, Dillon L. (2003) Quality in qualitative evaluation: a framework for assessing research evidence. London: Government Chief Social Researcher's Office, Prime Minister's Strategy Unit, Cabinet Office.

Swinkels A, Albarran JW, Means RI, Mitchell T, Stewart M. (2002) Evidence-based practice in health and social care: where are we now? *Journal of Interprofessional Care.* **16**(4): 335–47.

Van Driel M, Provoost S, Van Paepegem T, De Meyere M. (2003) *Op wetenschappelijke evidentie gebaseerde zorg: van theorie naar praktijk: een tweevoudige strategie.* Academia Press, Gent 57–73.

Van Duppen D, Aertgeerts B, Hannes K, Goossens F, Neirinckx J, Seuntjens L, Van linden A. (2007) Internet implementation of evidence based medicine during patient visits (online-on-the-spot). *Patient Education and Counseling.* **68**: 61–65.

Zaidi Z, Hashim J, Iqbal M, Quadri KM. (2007) Paving the way for evidence-based medicine in Pakistan. *J Pak Med Assoc.* **57**(11): 556–6.

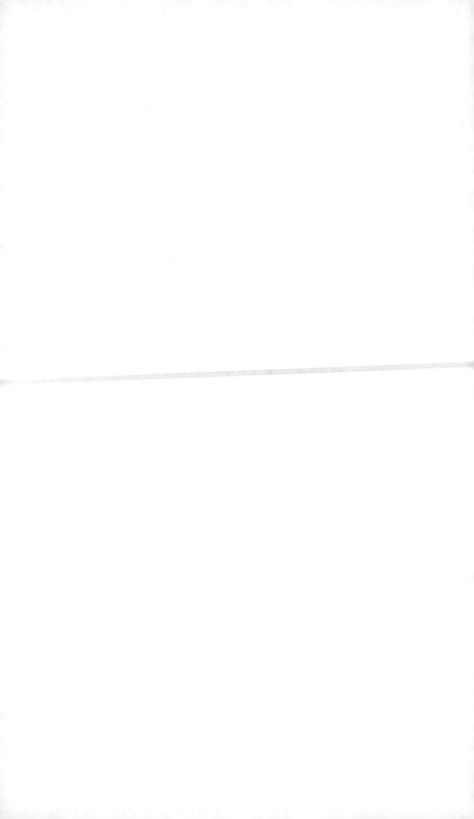

Chapter 3 Medicine taking for asthma: a worked example of meta-ethnography

Nicky Britten, PhD[1] and Catherine Pope, PhD[2]

[1]*Peninsula Medical School, University of Exeter, Exeter, Devon, UK*
[2]*University of Southampton, Southampton, UK*

Meta-ethnography is one of the most developed methods for synthesizing qualitative data and has been widely used, notably in educational, nursing, and other fields. Originally conceived by Noblit and Hare it seeks to develop a deliberately interpretative approach to synthesis by translating studies into one another thereby providing new interpretations. The aim of meta-ethnography is to arrive at an interpretation that is greater than that offered by the individual studies making up its constituent parts. It is the translative aspect that distinguishes meta-ethnography from other methods for qualitative synthesis. The worked example we use to illustrate this approach is on lay beliefs about medicine-taking for asthma, which was part of a broader synthesis which included other kinds of medicines for a range of other diseases and conditions. From the point of view of selecting papers for this synthesis, it was conceptual richness rather than methodological quality which characterized the "best" papers. The synthesis produced a line of argument which stated that a person's sense of identity is associated with the ways in which they perceive and use their medicines: those accepting the asthma identity will view medicines as an aid to normalization, while those not accepting this identity will view medicines as an obstacle to normalization. This synthesis revealed the inadequacy of the notion of compliance for understanding the ways in which people use their medicines. This is one example of a meta-ethnography that has contributed to conceptual development by producing new models, typologies, and concepts. Many more meta-ethnographies have been produced since then, aiming to contribute to the accumulation of qualitative research.

Synthesizing Qualitative Research: Choosing the Right Approach, First Edition.
Edited by Karin Hannes and Craig Lockwood.
© 2012 John Wiley & Sons, Ltd. Published 2012 by John Wiley & Sons, Ltd.

Introduction

Meta-ethnography is one of the most developed methods for synthesizing qualitative data and has been widely used, notably in educational, nursing, and other fields (Rice 2002; Jensen & Allen 1994; Paterson *et al.* 1998; Walters *et al.* 2004; Feder *et al.* 2006). It was developed by George Noblit and Dwight Hare, and outlined in their 1988 monograph for the Sage qualitative research methods series (Noblit & Hare 1998). The core features of meta-ethnography owe much to the applied research arena and philosophical orientation of its originators. Meta-ethnography was developed in response to the practical problem of dealing with the reports of different case studies on the same topic. The particular problem occupying Noblit and Hare at the time they developed meta-ethnography concerned the "desegregation ethnographies." These were a series of case studies undertaken between 1975–9 at the behest of a major US funding program, to investigate the implementation of policies to desegregate schools. Two attempts to summarize the available ethnographic case studies and aggregate the findings from the respective research reports failed to provide useful generalities for policymakers. This motivated Noblit and Hare to develop an approach that would allow them to synthesize these desegregation ethnographies successfully.

In designing this new method Noblit and Hare sought to develop a deliberately interpretative approach to synthesis, one that countered the prevailing positivist forms of knowledge synthesis which tended to emphasize the aggregation of evidence and favor quantitative systematic reviewing and statistical meta-analysis. Their desire to retain the interpretive essence of the ethnographic approach led them to decide that the synthesis method should be "grounded and comparative"(Noblit & Hare 1998, p. 23). In turn this led to their use of Stephen Turner's ideas about sociological explanation as translation (Turner 1980). It is this translative aspect which distinguishes meta-ethnography from other methods for qualitative synthesis. For Noblit and Hare the task of synthesis was not to provide generalization but to translate studies into one another thereby providing new interpretations. The aim of meta-ethnography is therefore to arrive at an interpretation which is greater than that offered by the individual studies making up its constituent parts. To use the definition cited by Noblit and Hare (1998) synthesis is an "activity or the product of an activity where some of the parts is combined or integrated into a whole ... [Synthesis] involves some degree of conceptual innovation of the parts as a means of creating the whole" (Nobilt & Hare 1998, p.16).

To summarize, the key features of meta-ethnography are as follows: it is a comparative approach to the synthesis of published research studies.

In Noblit and Hare's desegregation exemplar the studies were research reports which may be regarded as grey literature, whereas most of the subsequent applications use published research. It is interpretive rather than aggregative: the "meta" prefix signals an intention to "reveal analogies between accounts" (Noblit & Hare 1998, p.13) rather than averaging the results of several studies (as in meta-analysis). Finally the approach centers on the translation of qualitative studies into one another (Noblit & Hare 1998, p.25). Noblit and Hare's use of the term "meta-ethnography" arose from the nature of the case studies they originally synthesized; this terminology now identifies their method despite the fact that it has been used to synthesize other types of qualitative studies.

The method

Noblit and Hare suggest that the relationship between studies in a meta-ethnography may take one of three forms. Where the studies to be synthesized are directly comparable the synthesis takes the form of a *reciprocal translation*. This is an iterative process whereby the concepts from one study may be directly translated into the terms of another study. This translation may be taken further to develop what Noblit and Hare refer to as a *"lines-of-argument" synthesis*. This explores the similarities and differences between concepts proposed in the different studies, but moves towards a new interpretation, or "second-level" inference about what we can say about the whole based on the individual cases (this is akin to hypothesis generation).

In addition to these two forms, which are the most commonly found in the existing meta-ethnographic literature, Noblit and Hare speculate about a third form of synthesis called *refutational synthesis*. This is rooted in Kuhnian ideas about the importance of refutation in scientific progress, and suggests that studies that are oppositional require a specific form of interpretation and a distinct mode of synthesis. In this form the synthesis must take account of competing explanations and the relationship between them. There are, to our knowledge, no published examples of this form of meta-ethnography, beyond the two illustrations provided by Noblit and Hare in their monograph, which focus on a debate in the journal *Anthropology and Education Quarterly* and the controversy surrounding Freeman's critique of the work of Margaret Mead (1983).

Noblit and Hare outline seven phases which overlap and repeat in the development of a meta-ethnography. These are summarized below.

1 Getting started: identifying the research "interest."
2 Deciding what is relevant (mapping, searching, and selecting the literature).

3 Repeated reading of studies, extracting key concepts which are the "data" for the synthesis.
4 Determining the relationships between the studies.
5 Translating the studies into one another (a process that is analogous to constant comparison).
6 Synthesizing the translations by identifying concepts that can encompass those found on other studies.
7 Expressing the synthesis, typically in textual form but possibly in other presentational formats.

A worked example taken from the medicine-taking synthesis (Pound *et al.* 2005)

Noblit and Hare's work was first taken up by health service researchers over a decade after its original publication, and has been influential since then (Britten *et al.* 2002; Smith *et al.* 2005; Malpass *et al.* 2009). We are members of a larger team who were awarded a grant by the UK Health Technology Assessment (HTA) programme to appraise and synthesize qualitative health research for HTA using a meta-ethnographic approach (Campbell *et al.* in press). The team consisted of a group of experienced social scientists from a number of academic institutions in the UK. For this project we conducted two syntheses, one of lay beliefs about medicine-taking in chronic disease, and one about living with rheumatoid arthritis. These topics were chosen as they were topics familiar to the team, and about there were considerable bodies of published qualitative research available to synthesize. The worked example presented in this chapter draws from the medicine-taking synthesis (Pound *et al.* 2005) using a subset of the papers used for that synthesis. It therefore draws on the work of the entire team.

In the medicines synthesis, we adapted Noblit and Hare's seven phases to accommodate the number and diversity of the 38 papers in the synthesis. Specifically, we elaborated phases 4 and 5 into four new steps: organizing studies into medicine groups; translating studies into each other within medicine groups; determining how findings relate to each other within medicine groups and producing medicine maps; and determining how studies are related across medicine groups to produce an overall model of medicine-taking (Pound *et al.* 2005, p.140). This paper will focus on these four new steps, but first we describe how we tackled the first three phases of Noblit and Hare's model.

Phase 1: Identifying the research topic

The aim of the medicines synthesis was to synthesize the available qualitative research about lay experiences of medicine-taking, using meta-ethnography.

We knew that there were many published qualitative studies about this topic, and that it therefore constituted a suitable choice for the meta-ethnography. There are many other areas in which qualitative studies have been carried out but not synthesized: in other words, there is considerable scope for further syntheses.

Phase 2: Searching for studies

We carried out a literature search using the definition "Papers whose primary focus is patients' views of medicines prescribed and taken for the treatment of a long- or short-term condition" (Pound *et al*. 2005, p. 134). The study had to use both qualitative methods of data collection and analysis, and be published in English between 1 January 1992 and 31 December 2001. As the aim of this chapter is to illustrate the method rather than provide an up-to-date synthesis, we have not attempted to update the search. Details of the databases searched, the precise search strings used, and the search history are given in Pound *et al.*(2005). Of note here is the fact that, of the 43 papers identified, only half (22 papers) were identified electronically; the remaining 21 papers were identified by hand-searching journals.

Phase 3: Reading and appraising studies and identifying concepts

The papers identified during the literature search were appraised using modified Critical Appraisal Skills Programme (CASP) criteria for quality appraisal (CASP, 2006). Before using the CASP criteria, we screened the papers using the following screening questions:

1   Does the paper report on findings from qualitative research and did that work involve both qualitative methods of data collection and analysis?
2   Is the research relevant to the synthesis?

We defined "fatally flawed" papers as those papers for which the answer to the first question was "no." If the answer to either question was "no," the paper was excluded; if both answers were "yes," the appraisal could proceed. This involved answering questions about each paper in the following categories: aims, methodology, theoretical perspective, sampling, data collection, data analysis, research relations, data interpretation, transferability, relevance, and usefulness. The data recorded as a result of this appraisal process were both quantitative (yes/no answers) and qualitative (elaborating on these answers). A key part of this exercise was also to identify the main findings and concepts of each paper, which were recorded in an Access database. It was more efficient to do these two activities at the same time, as they both required detailed reading of all the papers. As a result of the appraisal exercise, 5 papers were excluded on the basis of the 2 screening questions, leaving a total of

38 papers to be synthesized. A further paper about asthma medications was excluded during the synthesis as it made no contribution to the synthesis. Despite having conducted detailed appraisals, we did not exclude papers on the basis of quality. We concluded that we would be unlikely to conduct such a detailed appraisal before conducting another synthesis. The advantage of carrying out some kind of appraisal is that it encourages careful and systematic reading of the papers. The consensus within the research team was that any future appraisal process could be much shorter, with just a few questions including the two screening questions to identify "fatally flawed" and irrelevant papers. The reason for this is that poor quality papers are likely to contribute less to the synthesis; rather than conduct a time-consuming quality appraisal process, it seems more useful to consider the value of the paper to the synthesis and exclude poor quality papers at the synthesis stage. While poor quality papers may contribute little to the synthesis, they may provide relevant descriptive data about the setting or participants for example. Malpass *et al.* (2009) categorized papers into four categories: key papers, satisfactory papers, irrelevant papers, and fatally flawed papers. We would endorse such an approach in future.

The concepts identified during the appraisal process were the raw data for the first stages of the synthesis. The distinction between concepts and themes is blurred, but we defined concepts as having some analytic or conceptual power, unlike more descriptive themes. Two independent reviewers extracted the concepts for each paper. In the few cases where a concept was only identified by one reviewer, it was included in the final list of concepts to ensure comprehensiveness. The key concept in the paper by Adams *et al.* (1997) was identity: this referred to the extent of respondents' acceptance or rejection of the identity of "asthmatic." Sub-concepts were personal identity, referring to the self, and social identity, referring to the "sum of an individual's group memberships, interpersonal relationships, social positions and statuses" (Adams *et al.* 1997, p. 199). Other aspects of identity were self-presentation, the stigma of asthma, and normalization (the attempt to lead a normal life). The key concept in the paper by Prout *et al.* (1999) was ordinariness: this reflected parents' stress on the ordinariness or normality of their child and his or her everyday life. A related concept was normalization, in this paper meaning the normalization of a child's symptoms as being very different from notions of asthma attacks. The key concept in the Buston and Wood paper (2000) was non-compliance, which provided the framework for a descriptive paper. The key concept in the paper by Walsh *et al.* (2000) was reciprocity, referring to the core reciprocal roles between the patient and the doctor including the rescued patient and the rescuing doctor. To exemplify the difference between themes and concepts, we would label the notion of "difficulty using inhaler" in the Buston and Wood paper as a theme, and the notion of "social identity" in the paper by Adams *et al.* as a concept. When extracting data about concepts, reviewers noted whether they were first order concepts (using respondents' words) or second order concepts (using authors' words) (Britten *et al.* 2002; Malpass *et al.* 2009). In this worked example, we used authors' labels for the concepts shown in Figure 3.1.

Phase 4: Organizing studies into medicine groups

Noblit and Hare's fourth stage involves consideration of how studies are related to one another. As the medicines synthesis included 38 papers, we chose to begin by grouping the papers on the basis of the medicines they referred to and the date of publication of the papers. This yielded seven "medicine groups:" anti-hypertensive medications (4 papers), medicines for HIV (11 papers), psychotropic medicines (6 papers), asthma medicines (4 papers), proton pump inhibitors (2 papers), studies on medicines in general (5 papers), and a group of medicines for miscellaneous illnesses (5 papers). In this chapter we will focus on the four asthma papers.

Phase 5: Translating studies into each other within medicine groups (reciprocal translations)

In the translation stage, we need to ask if concepts which have different labels are nonetheless describing the same idea. The translation of concepts for the medicines synthesis was carried out systematically within medicine groups by comparing each concept from each paper with all the other papers in turn. For example, paper 1 in the psychotropic medicine groups might have concepts X, Y, and Z. Paper 2 in the same group might have concept w (something new that was not found in paper 1), concepts x and y (similar to concepts X and Y in paper 1) and nothing like concept Z from paper 1. This would produce a synthesis of papers 1 and 2 as follows:

Concept w (from paper 2)

Concepts X and x (from papers 1 and 2)

Concepts Y and y (from papers 1 and 2)

Concept Z (from paper 1)

This synthesis of papers 1 and 2 would then be compared with paper 3 in the same way. Then the synthesis of papers 1, 2, and 3 would be compared with paper 4, and so on until all the studies within a single medicine group had been translated into one another. The labels used to describe the concepts could either come from one of the papers, as an author or second order concept, or could be chosen by the synthesizers (a third order concept). This process of translating concepts into one another is the process of "reciprocal

Factors influencing whether or not people take their medicine as prescribed
Acceptance of, or distancing from, asthma identity (A) – see opposite
Perceived effectiveness of (A, P, BW), fast acting nature of (P), convenience of (P), need for (BW) medicine
Whether medication supports ordinariness or stigmatizes (P, A)
Worries re steroids (A), s/effects (A, BW), dependency (A)
Lay evaluation/ experimentation re necessity of taking drugs (BW)

Are these factors influencing decision to take drugs OR incidental reasons why people don't take medicine as prescribed, or views of asthma meds?
Difficulty using inhalers (BW)
Inconvenience (BW)
Fast acting nature (P)
Convenience (P)

Children
The older children got the more autonomous they became in controlling meds (P)

Views of asthma meds:
Effective (P)
Fast acting (P)
Convenient (P)
Support ordinariness (P, Adam's Acceptors)
Inhalers allow targeting of precise quantities of medication to lungs, are small, unobtrusive, easy to use, allow rapid onset of drug action and reduce side effects (P)
Inhalers not seen as strong as inhaled and not systemic?(PP)
Asthma meds seen as preferable to avoidance/ (non- medical) preventive strategies (P)
Because asthma meds seen as so effective, hospital admission delayed even when serious (P)

Those who distanced selves from asthma identity: (A)
Viewed asthma as acute, not chronic (A)
Rejected identity of asthmatic, eg said had "bad chest" (A)
Downplayed severity – "only asthma"/ slight asthma (A, P, BW)
Denied, doubted they had asthma (A, P, W)
Did not take preventers (A) because: entailed acceptance of chronicity and asthma identity (A), fears
re steroids (A), s/effects (A), dependency (A)
Used reliever medicine (and more than optimum dose) (A) because: didn't fear dependency as only taken for symptom relief (A), seen to control condition (A)
Concealed use of inhalers because seen as stigmatizing and obstacle to normalization (A)
Operated policy of partial disclosure re their condition, preferring to present selves as normal (A)
Asthmatics viewed as weak and wimpy (A)
Have mechanical model of asthma as blocked tubes (A)
COULD THIS BOX BE PURPOSEFUL NON ADHERENTS/ ACTIVE MODIFIERS?

Characteristics of those who accepted asthma identity (A)
Incorporated asthma into lives (A)
Accepted chronicity of asthma (A)
Accepted need to take both preventive and reliever medication (A)
All carried reliever medication (A)
Did not like preventers because fears re steroids (A), s/effects (A), dependency (A)
Had tried to reduce use of preventers but unsuccessful so had accepted and routinized their use (A)
Medication seen as aid to normalization (A)
Operated policy of full disclosure; to deny asthma would be to deny important part of selves. Asthma identity not in conflict with other social identities. (A)
Asthmatics viewed positively (A)
Model of asthma is nearer medical understanding (A)
COULD THIS BOX BE PURPOSEFUL ADHERENTS/ ACTIVE ACCEPTERS?

Things that help people take medicines as prescribed
Relatives and friends reminding person to take meds (BW)
Establishing routines for taking meds (BW)
Negative experiences such as hospitalization (BW)

Figure 3.1 Asthma medicine map. Reproduced from Pound *et al.* Resisting Medicines: a synthesis of qualitative studies of medicine taking. *Social Science & Medicine* 2005; **61**(1): 133–155, 2005, with permission from Elsevier.

translation" as described by Noblit and Hare; we used this process as most of the papers were about similar issues with congruent findings. In particular, none of the findings refuted one another. We chose to use the term "concepts" rather than the term "metaphors" used by Noblit and Hare as we felt this provided a more accurate description of the material we were analyzing. Although the concepts lent themselves to reciprocal translation, one of the papers in the asthma medicine group was distinctive in employing a psychotherapeutic perspective to analyze the ways in which the doctor–patient relationship might influence the experience of taking asthma medicines (Walsh *et al.* 2002). Some of the concepts in this paper could be translated into those of the other papers in a reciprocal fashion, but others could not, largely because of the psychotherapeutic theories imposed on the data. This was in contrast to the concepts of "personal identity" and "social identity," based on symbolic interactionism, which emerged from the Adams *et al.* paper. The paper by Walsh *et al.* was included in the synthesis but remained somewhat detached from the others in the asthma group. If all the papers had been based on psychotherapeutic theories, it is likely that the concepts used by Walsh *et al.* would have translated into them. In other words, theories are likely to translate into each other if they are based on similar prior assumptions, although we have not tested this hypothesis.

Table 3.1 summarizes the initial process of translation of concepts for the four asthma papers. It includes data on the context of each paper, in terms of the nature of the sample, data collection, and setting. Three studies were carried out in general practice settings while the fourth was conducted in the context of a hospital asthma clinic. The table also shows the theoretical approaches taken by the authors of each paper, as this is often also relevant in the interpretation of concepts. Three of the papers were more or less explicit in using typologies to categorize respondents. Adams *et al.* (1997) clearly identified three groups: deniers, accepters, and pragmatists. Prout *et al.* (1999) did not categorize their respondents, while Buston and Wood (2000) were concerned with non-compliance, implicitly categorizing their respondents as non-compliers. Walsh *et al.* (2000) were also concerned with non-compliance and identified three patterns: denial, depression, and avoidance. Table 3.1 also shows the eventual synthesis categories, with the third order concepts of active accepters and active modifiers.

The table shows that the main concepts in the four papers were: identity (Adams *et al.* 1997), ordinariness (Prout *et al.* 1999), non-compliance (Buston & Wood 2000), and reciprocity (Walsh *et al.* 2000). The concepts of identity and ordinariness are linked; ordinariness can be seen as a component of identity. Both concepts include ideas of normalization. In considering the relationships between the concepts and interpretations of the

Table 3.1 Translation of concepts in four asthma papers

	Adams	Prout	Buston	Walsh
Journal/date	Social Science & Medicine 1997	Sociology of Health & Illness 1999	Family Practice 2000	British Journal of Medical Psychology 2000
Context				
Sample	30 adults prescribed prophylactic asthma medication	9 families with an asthmatic child	49 adolescents	35 patients prescribed bronchodilatory equipment
Data collection	In-depth home interviews	Intensive and repeated home interviews	In-depth home interviews	In-depth interviews
Setting	Single general practice in South Wales	Two general practice asthma clinics in North Midlands	Hospital asthma clinics in Greater Glasgow	Single general practice, location not stated
Theoretical approach (if any)	• Patient centered approach (p. 190) • Goffman's analysis of stigma (p. 192) • Symbolic interactionism (p. 199)	• Adaptation perspective (p. 140)	• Grounded theory approach (p. 135)	• PSORM (Procedural Sequence Object Relations) (p. 153) • SDR (Sequential Diagrammatic Reformulation) • Phenomenology • Psychotherapy
Categories of respondent	• Deniers/distancers • Accepters • Pragmatists		• Non-compliers	• Non-compliers • Denial • Avoidance • Depression

(Continued)

Table 3.1 (Continued)

	Adams	Prout	Buston	Walsh
Synthesis categories	• *Active accepters* • *Active modifiers*	• *Active accepters*	• *Active modifiers*	• *Active modifiers*
Concepts	IDENTITY (Social and personal) • Self-presentation • Stigma • Normalization • Attitudes to medication • Medication practice	ORDINARINESS • Normalization • Tolerability • Household management • Medication as central management strategy (p. 154)	NON-COMPLIANCE	RECIPROCITY • Rescuer • Rescued • Non-compliance
Interpretation	For the deniers, medication, particularly prophylactic medication, was viewed as a source of stigma and an obstacle to normalization: for the accepters it was an invaluable aid to normalization (p. 197)	Asthma medicines are attractive because they support ordinariness so effectively; non medicinal actions are unattractive because they undercut it so fundamentally (p. 157)	(Knowledge and non-compliance)	Potentially self harming health behaviors appear to be influenced by the subjectively experienced nature of the medical relationship (p. 162)
Citation of other papers in the synthesis	N/A – earliest paper	Adams	None	Adams

papers by Adams *et al.* and Prout *et al.*, it is worth noting differences in their sampling strategies. Adams *et al.* identified respondents from the database of a general practice, by including people who had been prescribed prophylactic asthma medication. Prout's sample was obtained via general practice asthma clinics. Thus the respondents in Prout's paper (or at least their parents, as the unit of analysis was families with an asthmatic child) could be assumed to have accepted the diagnosis of asthma; if not, it is unlikely that they would have attended asthma clinics. In contrast, respondents in Adams *et al.*'s study did not necessarily accept their diagnosis, and in fact several of them did not. Thus the respondents in Prout's study were comparable to Adams' accepters: for both of these groups, asthma medications helped them to achieve normalization (Adams *et al.* 1997) or ordinariness (Prout *et al.* 1999). The deniers in Adams' study had no counterparts in Prout's study; these were the people for whom asthma medication was stigmatizing and thus an obstacle to normalization. The paper by Buston and Wood is set within a biomedical framework of non-compliance, and is a largely descriptive paper with little conceptual development. While it provides some confirmation of the negative aspects of asthma medication, and a reference to denial of asthma (attributed to the adolescent respondents' earlier childhood years), it contributes little to the understanding of identity or ordinariness. As already noted, the paper by Walsh *et al.* is placed within a psychotherapeutic framework. Their description of denial corresponds to that in the other papers, but the analysis is placed within the context of the doctor–patient relationship, an issue mostly absent from the other papers. The issue of doctor–patient relationships arose in some of the other medicine groups, mostly in the context of patients withholding information about their actual medicine use from doctors for fear of being scolded. In other words, there was nothing in the rest of the medicines synthesis which could be translated into Walsh *et al.*'s concepts of "rescuer" and "rescued." Thus the two papers providing the most conceptual contribution to the asthma synthesis are those by Adams *et al.* and Prout *et al.*; this was because the concepts of identity and ordinariness were both analytically powerful and could be integrated to form more general interpretations (see below). In contrast, the concept of non-compliance was largely descriptive, and the concept of reciprocity (as explained by Walsh *et al.*) could not be translated into those of the other papers. In another synthesis containing more psychotherapeutically based papers, the paper by Walsh *et al.* could easily make a significant contribution.

Finally Table 3.1 shows the authors' interpretations of their findings for each paper, where given. Prout *et al.*'s interpretation that asthma medications are attractive because they support ordinariness is translatable into Adams *et al.*'s interpretation that for accepters, medication was an invaluable aid to normalization. Adams' further interpretation that medication was an obstacle to normalization for the deniers amplifies this argument.

Phase 6: Determining how findings relate to each other within medicine groups (producing "medicine maps")

The process of translation resulted in a textual synthesis for each of the medicine groups, in which concepts were described and related to the relevant papers. The next phase involved working out how the concepts related to one another. This was achieved by summarizing the concepts for each of the medicine groups so that they fitted on one page, and drawing the relationships between them. This resulted in a map for each of the medicine groups; these medicine maps summarized the key concepts, the way they translated into each other, and the relationships between them, for each of the groups. An early version of the asthma medicine map is shown in Figure 3.1. The letters A, P, BW, and W indicate the authors (Adams, Prout, Buston & Wood, and Walsh) of the paper each entry is taken from. The structure of the table reflects some of the concepts from the other medicine groups, as the maps were modified when compared with one another. By comparing the seven illness maps we could determine how the studies are related *across* illness groups, and we could use labels which applied across the whole synthesis. Thus the interim third order concepts of "purposeful adherents" and "purposeful non-adherents" became "active accepters" and "active modifiers" by the end of the synthesis.

Phase 7: Determining how studies are related across the medicine groups (model of medicine-taking)

On the basis of the comparison of medicine maps, a model was developed which encompassed the findings of all the papers in the synthesis (Figure 3.2). We considered using the model developed in one of the papers in the general medicines group (Dowell & Hudson 1997), but it could not account for all the papers in the synthesis. Our model describes the different ways in which people take medicines, which was not present in any of the individual papers but which is derived from them. The categories of "passive accepters," "active accepters," "active modifiers," and "rejecters" were all present in the asthma papers although the terminology is not identical. The particular issue of identity arising from the asthma papers is reflected in the model in relation to worries and concerns which cannot be dealt with by a process of evaluation, and which can lead to rejection of the medicine or to active modification. Those accepting the diagnosis of asthma may accept their medication passively or actively.

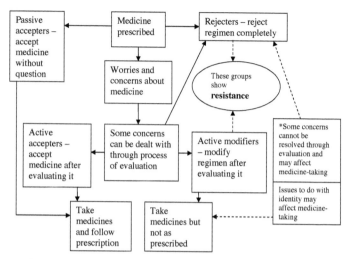

Figure 3.2 Model of medicine-taking. Reproduced from Pound *et al.* Resisting Medicines: a synthesis of qualitative studies of medicine taking. *Social Science & Medicine* 2005; **61**(1): 133–155, 2005, with permission from Elsevier.

The model provides a useful map of the synthesis process and may prove to be a useful model for understanding the route by which people decide whether and how to take their medicines. It shows that a diverse set of papers may be synthesized to create something new. However it only provides an overview without the detail.

Phase 8: Synthesizing translations across medicine groups (further conceptual development)

This final stage involved comparing the textual translations conducted for each of the medicine groups. This was achieved by reading and rereading each of the reciprocal translations, referring to the original papers where necessary, and analyzing the data thematically. This produced a line of argument synthesis as well as a reconceptualization of the findings. For the asthma papers, the line of argument was essentially the same as the interpretations given by Adams *et al.* (1997), supported by the those of Prout *et al.* In summary this line of argument states that a person with asthma's sense of identity is associated with the ways in which they perceive and use their medicines: those accepting the asthma identity will view medicines as an aid to normalization, while those not accepting this identity will view medicines as an obstacle to normalization. This line of argument did not make a major contribution to the whole synthesis as issues of identity did not arise in the other medicine groups in the same way. It constitutes a middle range theory which could be tested in other medicine groups or in other stigmatized conditions. For example, Malpass *et al.* refer to the "transformation of self-concept during treatment with antidepressants" (2009 p. 167), suggesting that issues of identity are relevant in other medicine groups as well as asthma medications.

The medicines synthesis as a whole showed that many lay people's response to medicines is best captured by the third order concept of resistance; in other words this concept was labeled by the synthesis team and not any of the respondents or authors (Pound 2005). This term encapsulated the way in which people take their medicines while also attempting to minimize their intake. This term also reflects people's active engagement with their medicines, and the ingenuity and energy they bring to dealing with them. In addition it suggests the ways in which people often conceal their actual medicine use from their doctors for fear of reprisals. This in turn reveals the power relations implicit in the traditional model of compliance, often experienced as coercive, particularly by those prescribed psychotropic medications. Thus the synthesis has helped reconceptualize lay experiences of medicine-taking by moving away from the concept of non-compliance and the focus on communication. Instead, the medicines themselves are seen as problematic. Patients are resisting the medicines and not necessarily the professionals, thus highlighting the fact that the issue may be more about drug safety and translation into patients' everyday lifeworlds rather than communication.

Conclusions

In this chapter we have demonstrated a worked example of the use of meta-ethnography as a method for synthesizing qualitative research. The synthesis resulted in a new model of medicine-taking, and the concept of resistance to encapsulate lay responses to medicines. This concept reveals the inadequacy of the notion of compliance for understanding the ways in which people use their medicines.

The challenges of this method include its time-consuming nature, which limits the number of studies which can be included in a single synthesis unless there is a large team of experienced qualitative researchers available to do the work. The medicines synthesis of which this worked example was a part took an experienced qualitative researcher (Pandora Pound) working part time, over 18 months to complete, with considerable additional input from the other team members. The work of Malpass *et al.* (2009) suggests that it is possible to identify in advance which key papers are likely to contribute most to the synthesis. If a systematic literature search produces large numbers of papers beyond the scope of the research team to synthesize, a reasonable compromise would be to limit the synthesis to key papers. In the worked example discussed in this chapter, the key papers were clearly those by Adams *et al.* and by Prout *et al.* Key papers are those which are conceptually rich, rather than merely descriptive. The concepts in key papers are likely to lend themselves to translation, and to form the basis of further interpretations and explanations which go beyond the settings of individual studies. From the point of view of selecting papers for a synthesis, it is conceptual richness rather than methodological quality which is likely to characterize the "best" papers.

Our first paper on meta-ethnography suggested that the purpose of qualitative synthesis was to build a cumulative knowledge base and to contribute to conceptual development (Britten 2002). In the course of conducting several meta-ethnographies since then, we have found that qualitative researchers tend not to cite each other's work. Thus if meta-ethnography contributes to bringing together diverse qualitative studies in the same field which have not built on each other's work, we suggest that it has contributed to the accumulation of qualitative research. The meta-ethnographies carried out by ourselves and others have also contributed to conceptual development by producing new models, typologies, and concepts (Campbell *et al.* 2003; Smith *et al.* 2005; Malpass *et al.* 2009).

Acknowledgements

The work reported in this chapter draws on the work of our collaborators Rona Campbell, Pandora Pound, Myfanwy Morgan, Gavin Daker-White, Roisin Pill, Lucy Yardley, and Jenny Donovan. It was funded by the UK Health Technology Assessment programme. Nicky Britten and Catherine Pope are partially supported by the UK National Institute of Health Research.

References

Adams S, Pill R, Jones A. (1997) Medication, chronic illness and identity: the perspective of people with asthma. *Social Science & Medicine.* **45**: 189–201.

Britten N, Campbell R, Pope C, Donovan J, Morgan M, Pill R. (2002) Using meta ethnography to synthesise qualitative research: a worked example. *Journal of Health Services Research and Policy.* **7**(4): 209–215.

Buston K, Wood S. (2000) Non-compliance amongst adolescents with asthma: listening to what they tell us about self-management. *Family Practice.* **17**: 134–138.

Campbell R, *et al.* (in press) Systematic appraisal and synthesis of qualitative research: evaluating meta ethnography. HTA Methodology Programme Grant, NCCHTA reference: 06/90/12. Details at http://www.hta.ac.uk/project/1563.asp [accessed 7 June 2011].

Campbell R, Pound P, Pope C, Britten N, Pill R, Morgan M, Donovan J. (2003) Evaluating meta-ethnography: a synthesis of qualitative research on lay experiences of diabetes and diabetes care. *Social Science and Medicine.* **56**: 671–84.

Critical Appraisal Skills Programme (CASP) (2006) 10 questions to help you make sense of qualitative research. http://www.phru.nhs.uk/Doc_Links/Qualitative%20Appraisal%20Tool.pdf [accessed 7 June 2011].

Dowell J, Hudson H. (1997) A qualitative study of medication-taking behaviour in primary care. *Family Practice.* **14**: 369–375.

Feder GS, Hutson M, Ramsay J, Taket AR. (2006) Women exposed to intimate partner violence: expectations and experiences when they encounter health care professionals: a meta-analysis of qualitative studies. *Arch Intern Med.* **166**: 22–37.

Freeman D. (1983) *Margaret Mead and Samoa: The Making and Unmaking of an Anthropological Myth.* Canberra: Australian National University Press.

Jensen LA, Allen MN. (1994) A synthesis of qualitative research in wellness-illness. *Qualitative Health Research.* **4**(4): 349–69.

Malpass A, Shaw A, Sharp D, Walter F, Feder G, Ridd M, Kessler D. (2009) "Medication career" or "Moral career"? The two sides of managing antidepressants: A meta-ethnography of patients' experience of antidepressants. *Social Science & Medicine.* **68**: 154–168.

Noblit G, Hare R. (1998) *Meta-ethnography: Synthesising Qualitative Studies.* Sage qualitative research methods series. Newbury Park CA, Sage.

Paterson BL, Thorne S, Dewis M. (1998) Adapting to and managing diabetes: Image: *Journal of Nursing Scholarship.* **30**(1): 57–62.

Pound P, Britten N, Morgan M, Yardley L, Pope C, Daker-White G, Campbell R. (2005) Resisting medicines: a synthesis of qualitative studies of medicine taking. *Social Science and Medicine.* **61**: 133–155.

Prout A, Hayes L, Gelder L. (1999) Medicines and the maintenance of ordinariness in the household management of childhood asthma. *Sociology of Health and Illness.* **21**: 137–162.

Rice EH. (2002) The collaboration process in professional development schools results of a meta-ethnography 1990–1998 *Journal of Teacher Education.* **53**(1): 55–67.

Smith L, Pope C, Botha J. (2005) Patients' help-seeking experiences and delay in cancer presentation: a qualitative synthesis. *Lancet.* **366**: 825–831.

Turner SP. (1980) *Sociological Explanation as Translation.* Cambridge: Cambridge University Press.

Walsh S, Hagan T, Gamsu D. (2000) Rescuer and rescued: applying a cognitive analytic perspective to explore the 'mis-management' of asthma. *British Journal of Medical Psychology.* **73**: 151–168.

Walters F, Emery J, Braithwaite D, Marteau T. (2004) Lay understanding of familial risk of common chronic diseases: a systematic review and synthesis of qualitative research. *Annals of Family Medicine.* **2**: 583–94.

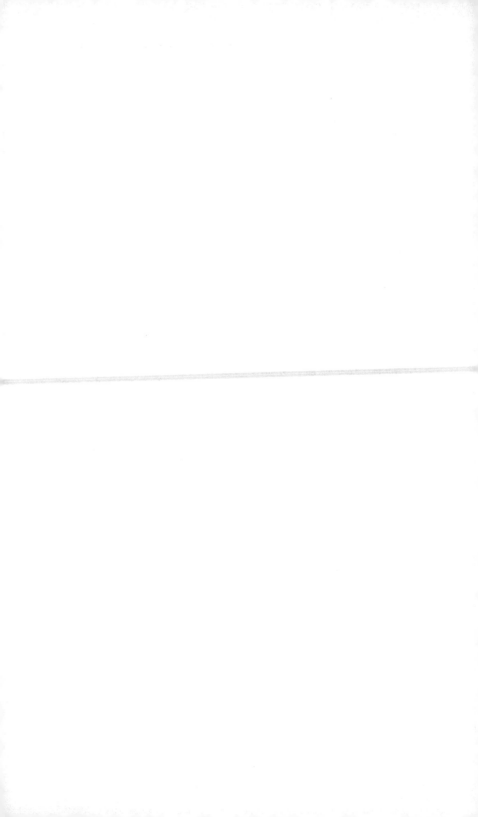

Chapter 4 The use of morphine to treat cancer related pain: a worked example of critical interpretive synthesis

Kate Flemming, PhD RN[1] and Elizabeth McInnes, PhD[2]

[1]*Department of Health Sciences, The University of York, York, UK*
[2]*Nursing Research Institute – Australian Catholic University and St Vincents and Mater Health Sydney, National Centre for Clinical Outcomes Research (NaCCOR), St Vincent's Hospital, Darlinghurst, NSW, Australia*

This chapter outlines an evolving approach, critical interpretive synthesis (CIS), to synthesizing a diverse body of qualitative and quantitative research literature. CIS shares characteristics with multilevel synthesis methods and is a useful synthesis technique for allowing findings from effectiveness literature to "interface" with the findings from qualitative research, thus enabling a synthesis between the findings from the two research paradigms. In this respect, it is a useful method for representing the views and perceptions of healthcare consumers about interventions that have been shown to be effective. A worked example of CIS illustrates the methods used in setting a question, searching the literature, quality appraisal, and analytical techniques.

Introduction

The aim of this chapter is to give an overview of critical interpretive synthesis (CIS) and a practical example of its use for synthesizing diverse studies using methods grounded in the interpretive tradition. This synthesis method is not as widely used as meta-ethnography and there are few practical examples. The main difference between meta-ethnography and CIS is that CIS evolved as a method to synthesize a large and diverse body of literature of different study designs around a particular topic. CIS can also be focused on critiquing the body of literature about a particular topic, examining what may have influenced proposed solutions to a problem (Dixon-Woods *et al.* 2006).

Synthesizing Qualitative Research: Choosing the Right Approach, First Edition.
Edited by Karin Hannes and Craig Lockwood.
© 2012 John Wiley & Sons, Ltd. Published 2012 by John Wiley & Sons, Ltd.

The chapter starts with an overview of mixed methods approaches to primary research and the principles of mixed methods which have informed the development of synthesis methods such as CIS, which embraces all types of evidence. A summary of the main features of CIS as developed by its founders is then given, followed by a worked example of CIS applied to a body of literature which includes effectiveness and qualitative research on the use of morphine to treat cancer-related pain. This is a new way of achieving a combined synthesis of diverse studies relating to a specific review objective, hence a detailed description of the methodological innovations and adaptations employed to undertake the synthesis of effectiveness and qualitative research is given. Differences and similarities between meta-ethnography and CIS are documented, because while CIS is a new method of synthesis it draws on some of the techniques of meta-ethnography, which is one of the more established methods for the synthesis of qualitative research (Pope & Mays 2006).

Mixed methods research

Traditionally there has been a widely held view that two methodological paradigms exist: qualitative and quantitative. Research has been conducted within the constraints of these paradigms with the differences apparent at a number of levels, from epistemology and theoretical framework, to methods and data collection techniques (Brannen 1992). Whilst the distinction between qualitative and quantitative research should be informed by epistemology and theory, it most commonly occurs at the level of method. The practicalities of research in healthcare mean that the supposed linear relationship from epistemology to method often becomes interrupted or distorted as different influences – such as funding sources, social organization, political orientations of research teams, and clinical speciality – exert forces over the research process (Bryman 1988). Consequently, decisions about choice of methods are influenced more by pragmatic, than epistemological, concerns and the value of using both methods to research a topic in order to understand both the micro and macro and the subjective and objective elements is more widely recognized (Bryman 1988). This has helped to spur the development of mixed methods not just in primary research but in relation to synthesizing diverse bodies of research from both quantitative and qualitative paradigms.

Circumstances of research and the need to represent the multifaceted nature of phenomena, rather than methodological or epistemological positions, are thus beginning to drive research agenda. By removing some of the distinctions between qualitative and quantitative research, a greater range of options for evaluating the complex nature of healthcare have become available. The consensus of their solely being two methodological paradigms is being challenged, along with the idea that these dichotomies represent good or bad, depending on the perspective of the researcher (Hammersley 1992). Each approach has its own strengths and weaknesses for conducting health-care research and this is sometimes behind the rationale for their integration (Bryman 1988). The conventional distinction of two opposing standpoints is being replaced by the idea of a range of positions which are located in more than one dimension, particularly as all research assumes there is a social reality which is amenable to observation (Hammersley 1992). Using a mixed methods approach for synthesis may also serve to "expose the tensions, map the diversity and communicate the complexity rather than reduce the literature to a simple, formulaic or universal solution" (Greenhalgh *et al.* 2005, p. 427).

Disassociating the epistemological roots of research from the methods and approaches used to conduct research has both advantages and disadvantages. The disadvantages are that research methods become detached from their epistemological and ontological beginnings and may loose their distinctiveness. There is a risk that researchers "pick and choose among the axioms of positive and interpretivist models" (Guba and Lincoln 2008, p. 266) without due regard for potential methodological incommensurability. The uncritical adoption of mixed methods approaches by researchers who are unaware of, or fail to appreciate, the underlying paradigmatic tensions, may lead to an assumption that the differences between them are merely technical rather than appreciating that the approaches were traditionally disparate (Sale *et al.* 2002). This lack of reflexive insight can lead to uncontextualized, descriptive accounts which lack theoretical engagement. Practically this can transfer into a mechanistic approach to mixed methods research which is self-referential and avoids questioning the production of knowledge (Fries 2009).

The main advantages of disassociation are thus: by taking a broad view of the epistemological assumptions which underpin qualitative and quantitative research, there is not disassociation from the roots but the adoption of a more pragmatic stance. This stance assumes that there is an empirical world that can be represented through research and that within each paradigm the appropriate application of mixed methodologies makes good sense (Guba & Lincoln 2008). In primary research there is acknowledgment that single methods, such as trials or qualitative research, may not satisfactorily address the complexity of decision-making in healthcare (Flemming 2007a).

The growing interest in using mixed methods research as a way of evaluating the complex nature of healthcare is also being emulated in the synthesis of research evidence. As highlighted elsewhere in this book, initial activity has concentrated on the development of methods to synthesize qualitative research. Much less attention has been paid to the development of methods to synthesize qualitative and quantitative research. The challenge has been to develop methods of synthesis which bring together effectiveness literature and qualitative research in a way that captures both systematic and interpretive methods of reviewing. Only a handful of exemplars exist. Completed syntheses mainly follow one of two broad approaches:

- *Multilevel synthesis* – Qualitative evidence (synthesis 1) and quantitative evidence (synthesis 2) are conducted as separate streams and the product of each synthesis is then combined (synthesis 3). A multilevel synthesis was used to answer the question: "What is known about the barriers to, and facilitators of, healthy eating among children aged 4–10 years?" (Thomas *et al.* 2004).

- *Parallel synthesis* – Qualitative evidence (synthesis 1) and quantitative evidence (synthesis 2) can be conducted as separate or linked reviews. The qualitative synthesis can then be used in parallel to aid the interpretation of the synthesized trials. Parallel synthesis was used to answer the research question "What are the facilitators and barriers to accessing and complying with tuberculosis treatment?" (Noyes & Popay 2007).

(*Source*: Noyes *et al.* 2008)

Both multilevel and parallel syntheses require a separate synthesis of qualitative and quantitative evidence. These are only synthesized with, or juxtaposed to, the synthesis of trials at a later point (Noyes *et al.* 2008). There is no interface between qualitative and quantitative research during the process of synthesis.

Critical interpretive synthesis

One approach which has been used to synthesize diverse bodies of literature that starts to combine qualitative and quantitative research is critical interpretive synthesis (CIS) (Dixon-Woods *et al.* 2006). CIS shares features of a mixed-methods approach in that it is a method of reviewing that integrates systematic review methodology with a qualitative tradition of enquiry, and was developed from meta-ethnography (Noblit & Hare 1988), discussed in Chapter 3. It explicitly allows the integration of qualitative and quantitative research and also theoretical papers. It will be seen from the worked example below that CIS is a form of combined synthesis that illustrates how qualitative research findings can address issues of relevance to the effectiveness literature. In this sense CIS shares characteristics with multilevel synthesis as described above.

Dixon-Woods' first example of a CIS addressed the issue of access to healthcare by vulnerable adults. The research question presented the authors with a diverse and wide ranging body of literature. The initial intention of the authors was to employ meta-ethnography as the method of synthesis for the review. The authors' experiences of working with a large and methodologically diverse sample of papers led them to refine and respecify a number of the concepts and techniques of meta-ethnography to enable the synthesis of the papers. Although the authors synthesized the findings of the studies included in the review, they were also interested in critiquing the body of literature. This new approach was termed critical interpretive synthesis and it is an approach to review that also facilitates critique of the literature and questioning of assumptions about concepts and methods that characterize the way in which a problem and solutions to the problem have been constructed. Dixon-Woods proposed that CIS was not purely a method for synthesis.

Importantly, Dixon-Wood's review demonstrated the potential for CIS to synthesize research papers from a wide range of qualitative and quantitative research methods. In order to further advance synthesis methods, the aim of the work presented in this chapter is to explore whether the processes of CIS could be adapted to specifically synthesize qualitative research with effectiveness research to answer a focused question that had arisen from clinical practice.

Methodology of CIS

Like meta-ethnography, CIS can enable the generation of theory and uses some of the tools of meta-ethnography. Unlike meta-ethnography, it has been used with a variety of study designs and generally uses a larger set of papers. CIS uses aspects of conventional systematic review methods but the typical staged and linear approach of systematic review is not used. For example, the authors of CIS (Annandale *et al.* 2007; Dixon-Woods *et al.* 2006) claim it is neither possible nor desirable to specify the review question in advance. Rather, the initial question should be modified in response to search results and findings and be used as a compass rather than an anchor. Purposive and theoretical sampling is used to add, test, and elaborate the emerging analysis. Searching proceeds concurrently with sampling. The point of termination is when the inclusion of new studies does not yield new insights (otherwise known as saturation). Papers are prioritized on the basis of relevance to the review objective rather than by study type or methodological criteria and formal quality assessment is not done. This means low-quality papers may be included on the basis of having high relevance. In common with other qualitative-based methods, complete transparency of process is not possible because of the interpretive elements used. This approach to selecting relevant research studies is used because the focus is on development of concepts and theory rather than on exhaustive summary of all data (Dixon-Woods *et al.* 2006). CIS also explicitly recognizes the voice of the "author" of the review and the partial nature of any account of the evidence (Annandale *et al.* 2007).

The primary output of a CIS is a synthesizing argument in which evidence from the included studies are integrated into a coherent framework, and this evidence has been transformed into a new conceptual form called a synthetic construct (Annandale *et al.* 2007). A network of constructs based on the studies and relationships between constructs is created. Arguably, this is similar to "line-of-argument" in meta-ethnography. Like other qualitative-based synthesis methods, the synthesizing process enables CIS to develop understandings that are more insightful and conceptual than more descriptive forms of thematic analysis. Contradictions between studies are descriptively considered as part of the analysis that produces the synthesizing argument.

CIS is claimed to provide an alternative to existing synthesis methods by having tested the inclusion of a diverse body of literature (both qualitative and quantitative) and by the use of critical inquiry. Its originators claim it is most suitable for broad questions with diverse literatures and where the aim is to generate a synthesizing argument (mid-range theory). In addition, part of CIS may be to critically examine the included literature on a topic by questioning the epistemological and normative assumptions on which the literature draws, and examine the construction of concepts such as healthcare access (Annandale *et al.* 2007). This means the research literature is looked at as "*an object of scrutiny*" examining how the problem/issue has been represented, constructed, and reported in the research literature, as well identifying the epistemological assumptions on which the literature draws (Annandale *et al.* 2007).

As shown in Table 4.1, while the key stages are much the same as for meta-ethnography, there are some differences. CIS analysis leads to the generation of a synthesizing argument organized around a set of central concepts which are termed synthetic constructs, but which can be considered as equivalent to the "third-order constructs" identified in meta-ethnography. Synthetic constructs refer to a new conceptual form that has come about through a process of transformation of the evidence (Annandale *et al.* 2007). Again, similar to meta-ethnography, a network of constructs based on the studies and relationships between constructs is created. Contradictions between studies are descriptively considered as part of the analysis that produces the synthesizing argument.

Table 4.1   Comparison between the phases of meta-ethnography and critical interpretive synthesis

Phase of meta-ethnography	Critical interpretive synthesis
Phase 1: Getting started Identifying an intellectual interest that qualitative research might inform	Identifying an area of clinical interest
Phase 2: Deciding what is relevant to initial interest Searching for studies to be included	Searching for studies
Phase 3: Reading the studies Repeated re-reading of studies to identify concepts/metaphors	*Understanding the paper in relation to itself* Reading the paper to develop an understanding of its position and context prior to comparing it to others. This was not identified as a separate process in Dixon-Woods's description of CIS
Phase 4: Determining how the studies are related Determining the relationships between the studies	
Phase 5: Translating the studies into one another Comparison with metaphors/concepts in one study with those in other studies. Translations can be reciprocal, refutational, or form a "line-of-argument"	*Translating studies into one another* The concepts, themes and metaphors used by authors are identified and translated from one study into another to produce a reduced account of the content and context of all studies
Phase 6: Synthesizing translations Secondary translation (not always possible) when translations can encompass those of other accounts producing third order constructs?	*Synthesizing translations* Translations compared to determine if either the translations and/or concepts to encompass those of other accounts. Through **reciprocal translation analysis (RTA)** evidence can be transformed into a new conceptual form called **synthetic constructs**

(Continued)

Table 4.1   (Continued)

Phase of meta-ethnography	Critical interpretive synthesis
Phase 7: Expressing the synthesis Communication of the findings from the meta-ethnographic synthesis in a form appropriate for the audience	Evidence from across studies is integrated into a comprehensible theoretical framework called a **synthesizing argument**. This represents the network of synthetic constructs and explains the relationships between them, with the aim of providing "more insightful, formalised and generalisable ways of understanding a phenomenon" (Dixon-Woods *et al.* 2006a p. 5).

A worked example of critical interpretive synthesis

The worked example described here is one in which the process of CIS is applied to a body of literature on the use of morphine to treat cancer-related pain. A detailed description of the methodological innovations employed to undertake the synthesis of effectiveness and qualitative research are described, specifically the adaptations made to CIS that enabled this.

The main difference between the methods of the CIS in this section and the earlier example from Dixon-Woods is that what is described here does not involve a "critique" of the literature. In their review of "Access to Health Care by Vulnerable Adults," Dixon-Wood *et al.* describe critique as:

"A key feature of this process [*critique*] that distinguishes it from some other current approaches to interpretive synthesis (and indeed of much primary qualitative research) was its aim of being critical: its questioning of the ways in which the literature had constructed the problematics of access, the nature of the assumptions on which it drew, and what has influenced its choice of proposed solutions. Our critique of the literature was thus dynamic, recursive and reflexive, and, rather than being a stage in which individual papers are excluded or weighted, it formed a key part of the synthesis, informing the sampling and selection of material and playing a key role in theory generation." (p. 6)

Rather, in the example described here, CIS is principally used to synthesize a large and diverse body of evidence comprising qualitative and quantitative research (not including theoretical papers) in order to construct a body of evidence about effective morphine use in cancer patients that reflects the views of patients, carers, and healthcare professionals. It was not the aim to examine, for example, what has influenced the choice of and dominance of morphine for cancer pain, nor to deconstruct the research that has supported the use of morphine. Purposive and theoretical sampling of the literature was also not done because a relatively small set of papers (n = 15) met the inclusion criteria. Reciprocal translation analysis was used in this worked example; in the earlier published CIS work, this analysis technique was tested but found difficult to use with a large number of papers of diverse methodologies.

Question development

The approach to question formulation in meta-ethnography involves "identifying an intellectual interest that qualitative research might inform" (Noblit & Hare 1988, p. 26), after which relevant points are identified. This differs greatly to the stance to question formulation taken in systematic reviews of effectiveness when the question is identified a priori and becomes the anchor for the review from which its parameters are set. Within CIS, question formulation reflects the approach taken by meta-ethnography, with the posing of a question that identifies an area of interest, not a specific hypothesis. Whilst there are no formal requirements for the formation of a research question, pragmatically the identification of the population of interest, perhaps the setting, and additional contextual factors will guide the structure of the question and subsequent literature searches.

The focus of the synthesis was the use of morphine to treat cancer-related pain. Two syntheses of the effectiveness of morphine: a Cochrane Systematic Review – Oral Morphine for Cancer Pain – a systematic review of 54 randomized controlled trials reporting the analgesic effect of oral morphine (Wiffin & McQuay 2007); and the European Association of Palliative Care (EAPC) recommendations for the use of morphine and alternative opioids to treat cancer pain (Hanks *et al.* 2001), were the starting point of the review. The systematic review findings and guideline recommendations were chosen pragmatically as examples of the effectiveness literature that might prove feasible to be synthesized with qualitative research. The aim of the synthesis was to determine the way in which the recommendations for morphine use arising from the effectiveness literature reflected the perceptions of patients, carers, and healthcare professionals of using morphine, and how the combination of these may impact on practice.

Methods of searching

Strategy for searching

The focus of this review was to determine whether CIS could be used to synthesize qualitative and quantitative research answering a reasonably focused clinical question. As the quantitative literature had been identified in the form of an effectiveness review and clinical guideline, the aim of searching was to identify qualitative research relevant to the review aim. Hence in this example we concentrate only on the search strategy for the qualitative studies. As a result the review used protocol-driven, electronic search strategies which have been demonstrated as effective for finding qualitative research for questions with a clear focus (Flemming & Briggs 2007). Previously reviews using CIS have undertaken structured protocol driven searching, but have combined this with a more "organic" approach of hand-searching, reference-chaining, and consultation with experts (Dixon-Woods *et al.* 2006) due to the broader research question and the large quantity of literature involved. As a body of work in CIS develops it may be that different approaches to searching for qualitative research are undertaken depending on the topic of the review. For this review, a search strategy was written which combined search terms for morphine (based on those used by the Cochrane Pain Palliative and Supportive Care Group for oral morphine for cancer pain review) with broad-based terms to identify qualitative research. The combination of a three-line search strategy using broad qualitative search terms (shown in lines 39–41 of the search strategy in Table 4.2) with clinical terms has been shown to be as effective as the combination with a longer 48-line strategy using free text terms describing qualitative research (Flemming & Briggs 2007). This approach to searching was replicated in this review.

The search was run in Medline and was refined iteratively (Sindu & Dickson 1997) through key terms identified from relevant papers in the preliminary search being incorporated into a revised search strategy. The search was adapted for and run in OvidSP Medline (1950–2008), Cinahl (1982–2008), Embase (1980–2008), PsychINFO (1967–2008), HMICC (Health Management Information Consortium, May 2008) and Web of Science SSCI (1956–2008). Electronic searching was supplemented by informal methods of: reference-chaining; hand-searching of journals known to publish qualitative research in palliative care; and contact with experts.

Inclusion and exclusion criteria
The inclusion criteria for obtaining full text of an article were: described the results of empirical qualitative research relevant to the review question; referred to the use of morphine or other opiates to treat cancer related pain; was published in English.

Table 4.2 Search strategy. Reproduced from Flemming K. 'Synthesis of quantitative and qualitative research: an example using Critical Interpretive Synthesis', Journal of Advanced Nursing 2010; 66(1):201–217, 2010, with permission from John Wiley & Sons Ltd.

1 Morphine$.mp.
2 Morphine.mp
3 Delayed-action-preparation$.mp.
4 tablets-enteric-coated.mp.
5 (1 or 2) and (3 or 4)
6 (Morphine adj5 (sustained adj release)).mp.
7 (morphine adj5 sustained-release).mp.
8 (morphine adj5 (controlled adj release)).mp.
9 (morphine adj5 controlled-release).mp.
10 (morphine adj5 (immediate adj release)).mp.
11 (morphine adj5 immediate-release).mp.
12 (morphine adj5 (modified adj release)).mp.
13 (morphine adj5 modified-release).mp.
14 (morphine adj5 (extended adj release)).mp.
15 (morphine adj5 extended-release).mp.
16 (morphine and (MST or SRM or IRM or MSS or MSC or MOS or MIHR)).mp.
17 (morphine and contin).mp.
18 (morphine adj5 (oral adj solution)).mp.
19 kadian.mp.
20 kapanol.mp.
21 administration-oral.mp
22 1 or 2 or 5 or 6 or 7 or 8 or 9 or 10 or 11 or 12 or 13 or 14 or 15 or 16 or 17 or 18 or 19 or 20
23 ((oral-administration or oral) adj administration).mp.
24 (oral adj route).mp.
25 (oral adj5 morphine).mp.
26 oral-morphine.mp.
27 23 or 24 or 25 or 26
28 22 and 27
29 neoplasm$.mp.
30 cancer$.mp.
31 neoplasm.mp.
32 29 or 30 or 31
33 Pain.mp.
34 pain-measurement.mp.
35 pain-threshold.mp.
36 pain$.mp.
37 34 or 35 or 36
38 28 and 32 and 37
39 findings.af.
40 interview$.af or interviews/
41 qualitative.af.
42 or/39-41
43 38 and 42

Results of searching

The electronic searches yielded a total of 2,886 records. Abstracts of 225 records were retrieved. Of these, 30 full text articles were obtained. A further 10 records were identified through informal searching methods, of which 7 were obtained in full text. In a synthesis of qualitative research exploring patient experience of living with leg ulceration, the reviewers found that it was personal knowledge of papers that led to identification of papers which had been excluded when screened by title alone (Flemming & Briggs 2007).

Thirty-seven full text papers were therefore retrieved to determine whether they matched the inclusion criteria. At this point eighteen papers were excluded, for two main reasons: papers were not reports of qualitative research, or papers did not deal explicitly with issues related to cancer pain or the use of opiates. Nineteen qualitative papers, reporting on fifteen studies were included (Figure 4.1). The studies that were reported in more than one paper were included, as different populations were represented within each paper, for example views' of patients, healthcare professionals, and carers were reported in separate publications.

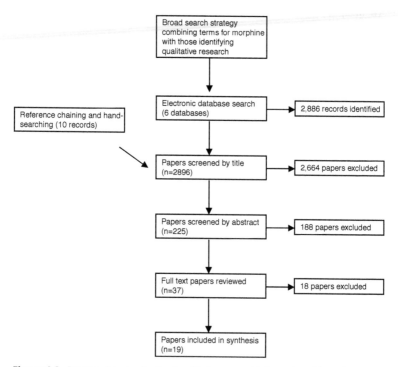

Figure 4.1   Process of study selection (qualitative research). Reproduced from Flemming K. 'Synthesis of quantitative and qualitative research: an example using Critical Interpretive Synthesis', Journal of Advanced Nursing 2010; 66(1):201–217, 2010, with permission from John Wiley & Sons Ltd.

If there had been a large number of papers, the recommended approach is to draw on the sampling techniques of primary qualitative research (Dixon-Woods *et al.* 2006). For example, Dixon-Woods *et al.* (2006) report that at the outset of their review they used purposive sampling to select papers that were highly relevant to the review aim. The authors later used theoretical sampling of additional papers to add, test, and elaborate their emerging analysis. Theoretical saturation then was used to determine the point of saturation of their analysis and to cease including additional papers.

Determination of quality

Appraisal of the quality of qualitative research remains a contentious issue, reflecting some of the tensions apparent in qualitative research itself (Dixon-Woods *et al.* 2007a). The most common approach to appraisal has been in the form of structured checklists. In general, where quality appraisal has been undertaken within syntheses of qualitative research (approximately 50% of reviews, Dixon-Woods *et al*, 2007b) papers have not been excluded on the grounds of quality. Where papers have been deemed as inferior but included, it has been asserted that they can contribute to theoretical development of the synthesis topic, although often provide "less "weight' within a synthesis (ie, contribute less) than those papers deemed of better quality (Noblit & Hare 1982; Atkins *et al.* 2008; Dixon-Woods *et al.* 2006; Hawker *et al.* 2002). Quality appraisal was undertaken in this review in order to record the quality of the identified qualitative research against predetermined criteria. It is acknowledged, however, that quality appraisal may become an exercise of judging the quality of the published report, rather than being an evaluation of the research process itself (Sandelowski & Barroso 2002; Atkins *et al.* 2008).

A quality appraisal checklist was used consisting of nine questions, each of which has four sub-categories as shown in Table 4.3 (Hawker *et al.* 2002). A protocol provides descriptors for each category. The system allows for the calculation of a summed score of methodological quality which ranges from 9 (very poor) to 36 (good) and enables transparency as the descriptors enable an explicit scoring of each paper. This affords the appraisal of qualitative research some elements of transparency associated with the appraisal of RCTs, and has been shown to make reviewers more explicit about the reasons for their judgments (Dixon-Woods *et al.* 2007a). Each paper was assessed for quality by the author. A cross-section of the papers was second-checked by another author for accuracy. No disagreements occurred.

Most papers were considered to be of reasonable methodological quality, with scores ranging from 19–34, and all were included. The lowest scoring paper (Wheeler 2005) was an "outlier" (the next lowest score being 24) but was included due to its relevance to the synthesis topic. Examining the contribution

Table 4.3 Quality appraisal checklist. Reproduced from Flemming K. 'Synthesis of quantitative and qualitative research: an example using Critical Interpretive Synthesis', Journal of Advanced Nursing 2010; 66(1):201–217, 2010, (using data from Hawker *et al* 2002), with permission from John Wiley & Sons Ltd.

	Good	Fair	Poor	Very poor	Comment
1 Abstract and title					
2 Introduction and aims					
3 Method and data					
4 Sampling					
5 Data analysis					
6 Ethics and bias					
7 Findings and results					
8 Transferability/generalizability					
9 Implications and usefulness					
Total					

this paper made to the development of synthetic constructs and the synthesizing arguments at the end of the process confirmed that this decision was correct.

Data extraction

All papers were subject to data extraction. A pro-forma was devised to enable the summary of information on the aim of the research, participants, methodology, methods of data collection, methods of analysis, and key results in the form of authors' main findings and participant verbatim quotes. The extent to which these data could be recorded was dependent on the clarity of reporting within papers. A summary of this information was then transferred into the qualitative software Atlas-Ti to ensure that all findings remained linked to the context from which they were drawn. The role of data extraction within the synthesis of qualitative research requires formal evaluation (Dixon-Woods *et al.* 2006). Using a summary of the extracted information as a contextual link in Atlas-Ti was found to be helpful in this instance.

Conducting the synthesis

Prior to this review CIS had only been used with a large diverse body of primary research. It had not been used to synthesize existing systematic reviews with primary qualitative research with a specific focus. It was anticipated that some of the processes involved in CIS may require adaptation given the unique starting point of this review. One example of this is that the process of RTA was found to be impossible when synthesizing a diverse and large body of literature. It was acknowledged by Dixon-Woods *et al.* that this does not make RTA redundant within CIS, but it was not of value with the body of literature they were dealing with. As this review of morphine use contained only 19 related qualitative research papers, it was considered appropriate to try to use RTA and evaluate its role within CIS.

Translating the quantitative and qualitative research into one another

Integrating the findings of qualitative and quantitative studies
The establishment of methods to allow the effectiveness literature to "interface" with the qualitative research was essential to this review, to enable a synthesis between the findings from the two research paradigms. Taking the principles of reciprocal translation analysis, which "protect the particular, respect holism, and enable comparison" (Noblit & Hare 1988, p. 28), the findings of the Cochrane Systematic Review and the EAPC guidelines were read and used as a framework to guide the extraction of findings from the qualitative research papers. Using a framework approach enabled the valuable aspects of the effectiveness literature; the notion of "what works and when to use it," not only to be protected, but to be compared with the "what are the implications of this" arising from the qualitative research. An RTA is deemed effective when it maintains the central concepts of one account in relation to key concepts in other accounts. The aim of the framework was to ensure that none of the key aspects of either the quantitative or the qualitative research was lost at the point of interface.

The method used to achieve this was an integrative grid. Along the top of the grid were the findings from the Cochrane Review and statements from the EAPC guidelines (20 columns). Each row of the grid represented a qualitative research paper (19 rows). The interface between qualitative and quantitative research occurred in the cells of the grid, which were populated by findings from the qualitative research. This showed how the qualitative findings fitted with the recommendations from the quantitative research, and supported the development of a coding framework. A sample of the grid is shown in Table 4.4.

Using the grid enabled a visual guide to the weighting of the qualitative research in relation to the quantitative. For example the first column entitled "Opioid of first choice is morphine" (representing EAPC recommendation one) was highly populated with contributions from all but three qualitative studies, whereas other columns, often relating to more technical findings from the effectiveness data such as "recommendations for oral to intravenous conversion rates for morphine," contained no data. This illustrated how the qualitative research findings addressed issues of relevance to the effectiveness literature, which has not been the case in other combined syntheses (Thomas & Harden 2008).

Table 4.4 Sample from within the integrative grid. Reproduced from Flemming K. 'Synthesis of quantitative and qualitative research: an example using Critical Interpretive Synthesis', Journal of Advanced Nursing 2010; 66(1):201–217, 2010, with permission from John Wiley & Sons Ltd.

	Opioid of first choice is morphine	If pain returns on a regular basis, regular dose should be increased and rescue medication taken	For patients on normal release medication a double dose should be taken at bedtime	Successful pain management requires adequate analgesia without adverse effects
Coyle 2004	• Morphine is viewed as positive to relieve pain • Good analgesia leads to a sense of control	• Poorly controlled pain is interpreted as worsening disease • Unlimited analgesia is required for a comfortable death		• Adverse effects are a burden • Cognitive side effects lead to "loss of self" • Opioids are a burden because of side effects
Ersek *et al.* 1999	• Need to prove pain to get analgesia • Patients took opioids regularly to improve functioning • Side effects are tolerated		• Patients wake at night in pain as they can't afford sustained release preparations	• Functionality more important than pain relief • Adverse effects are a deterrent • Analgesic use altered due to side effects • Side effects seen as a sign of addiction

(Continued)

Table 4.4 (Continued)

	Opioid of first choice is morphine	If pain returns on a regular basis, regular dose should be increased and rescue medication taken	For patients on normal release medication a double dose should be taken at bedtime	Successful pain management requires adequate analgesia without adverse effects
Johnston-Taylor et al. 1993	• Morphine works so it gets taken despite side effects	• Patients had conflict over management of opioids, what, when how to take?		• Negative connotations associated with morphine use because of side effects • Carers have concerns over side effects and addiction • Nurses concerns over side effects
Reid et al. 2008	• Increasing requirement for morphine signified impending death • Painkillers may hasten or signify death • Morphine is a last resort • Morphine is frightening • Doses of morphine will only increase • Opioids cause deterioration • No choice but to commence opioids when pain is severe			• High doses of morphine cause sedation and death • Trade-off between pain relief and loss of function

Secondary translation of qualitative studies

As the integrative grid developed, it became apparent that the qualitative research addressed issues wider than those specifically mapped to the effectiveness literature and these findings needed to be incorporated into the overall synthesis. As a result a secondary translation of qualitative studies was undertaken using the coding framework developed through the grid. Computer software "Atlas-Ti," designed for qualitative analysis of large bodies of text, was used in this translation. Findings from the primary qualitative research were entered verbatim into Atlas-Ti as "primary documents". Findings were classed as themes and sub-themes reported by researchers in the "results" or "findings" section of primary papers. This second extraction of findings was more extensive than the first.

The findings were initially coded in accordance with the identified framework. The codes were listed in the "code manager" function of Atlas-Ti and were directly traceable back to their primary research source. Other findings not picked up by the framework coding were then identified and coded. This ensured that the findings from the Cochrane Review and EAPC recommendations directed the coding, but other contextual qualitative findings were incorporated into the synthesis. Some findings became codes in themselves, whereas others became codes in combination with others. The codes were refined and extended as each study was added to the framework. As a result RTA became a two-stage process. As the synthesis had the explicit aim of integrating specific effectiveness data with related qualitative research, this first stage of the synthesis—creating an integrative grid— does not feature in CIS, but can be seen as a variant of RTA. By producing an integrative grid, the key findings and recommendations for practice from the effectiveness research were directly compared with the relevant concepts and metaphors from the qualitative research. Theoretically it would be possible for the RTA to be completed in one phase if all the findings from the qualitative research were incorporated into the integrative grid, although it is unlikely that such a perfect fit will occur between qualitative and quantitative research. Therefore a second stage of RTA is likely to be required in most instances.

Development of synthetic constructs and synthesizing arguments

The findings from a CIS are expressed in the form of a synthesizing argument. This is developed from synthetic constructs and the findings of primary research, and is the process by which CIS becomes distinct from meta-ethnography.

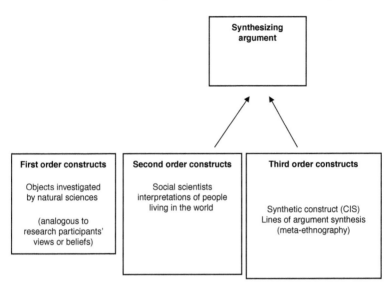

Figure 4.2 The relationship of a synthesizing argument to first, second, and third order constructs.

Researchers who have developed meta-ethnographic methods have built on the notion of first and second orders of constructs (Schutz 1973) by representing second order constructs as translations that are synthesized into "third order" constructs and labeled a "lines of argument" synthesis (Figure 4.2). Examples of lines of argument syntheses arising from meta-ethnographies include: identifying factors that influence adherence to TB treatment (Munro *et al.* 2007); the "strategic non-compliance" used by people with diabetes to manage their condition (Campbell *et al.* 2003); the identification of "forms of medicine taking" by patients (Britten *et al.* 2002).

There are limitations associated with the role of Schutz's order of constructs in meta-ethnography. Many of the interpretations identified as second order constructs are descriptive in nature and appear subjective. This is a product of the poor quality of the conduct and/or reporting of some qualitative research and can cause difficulty in undertaking translations and creating third order constructs (Atkins *et al.* 2008).

Within CIS the notion of the meta-ethnographic lines-of-argument synthesis is developed, with the output from this phase of synthesis represented as a "synthesizing argument" consisting of both second and third order constructs. A synthesizing argument is not analogous to a "third order" construct, but forms an amalgamation of author interpretations and synthetic constructs (Figure 4.2). Consequently CIS does not make a precise distinction between

Table 4.5   Synthetic constructs. Reproduced from Flemming K. 'Synthesis of quantitative and qualitative research: an example using Critical Interpretive Synthesis', Journal of Advanced Nursing 2010; 66(1):201–217, 2010, with permission from John Wiley & Sons Ltd.

Synthetic construct	Number of contributing codes
The role and influence of the healthcare professional in the management of pain	55
Management of pain by the patient	46
The meaning of pain	37
The role of carers	33
End of life	31
The influence of cancer pain on patients and carers	30
Views on morphine and opioids	24
The meaning of cancer	23
Addiction, abuse, and tolerance concerns	19
Control	13
Adverse effects of opioids	13
Trade-off/balancing act	12
Spirituality and religion	9
Parenteral opioids	3

second and third order constructs and allows rich description of phenomena in primary studies to influence the format and shape of the synthesizing argument.

The synthesis produced 14 synthetic constructs from 255 codes created through the RTA (Table 4.5). Constructs were developed by examining codes to identify unifying ideas. Some of the codes were clearly identifiable as forming a construct due to their uniform nature, "Adverse effects of opioids" being one example. Other constructs were formed by collapsing groups of codes into a renamed construct. Some codes featured in more than one synthetic construct. For example the code "fear of dying in pain" featured within the synthetic constructs "the influence of cancer pain on patients," "meaning of pain," and "end of life."

The development of the synthesizing arguments was driven by the initial focus of the synthesis with the findings from the effectiveness data being constantly compared with theoretical developments. This reflected the iterative process used during the formation of the codes and subsequently the synthetic constructs. Four synthesizing arguments were developed from the synthetic constructs and the coding arising from the processes of RTA:

- opioids and opioid concern
- using opioids is a balancing act and a trade-off
- the existential meaning of cancer and cancer pain
- the inter-subjectivity of pain.

A mediating factor that ran through all of the synthesizing arguments was the synthetic construct of "control" and as such was presented as an overarching part of the synthesis. Control of cancer related pain is at the core of this synthesis; it was apparent as a second order construct and formed a synthetic construct. The essence of "control" was that patients can perceive cancer pain to be enormous, exceeding all sense of control. Achieving pain control was essential to patients' sense of self-control. It made sense that "control" became a mediating factor for all the synthesizing arguments, rather than feeding into each of them individually.

Producing discrete synthesizing arguments was difficult, with some synthetic constructs contributing to more than one synthesizing argument. This has been a feature of other critical interpretive syntheses. The CIS of access to healthcare reports how the synthetic constructs developed were linked, with the synthesizing argument being developed around one core construct of candidacy (Dixon-Woods *et al.* 2006). What drove the development of separate synthesizing arguments within this CIS was the perceived need to define the discrete characteristics of the synthesizing arguments, rather than just report common features. It was considered that this was important in driving the theoretical developments that could influence the clinical practice of using morphine to treat cancer-related pain. There is no clear indication at this point in the development of CIS that discrete synthesizing of synthetic constructs and synthesizing arguments is possible or indeed desirable. It will only be with continued use of the method that clarity will emerge.

Conclusion

This chapter has presented a background to the development of research methods inclusive of qualitative and quantitative research methods and linked this to the development of synthesis methods that include both qualitative and quantitative research studies. CIS is an evolving synthesis method that has extended and adapted the methods of meta-ethnography to include a large and diverse literature on specific topics. The worked example here has used CIS to provide an analysis of findings from an effectiveness review, national guidelines, and qualitative studies but has used the technique of RTA as part of the analysis repertoire. Future work in this area may concentrate on how a synthesis looks if only the data that "interface" between qualitative and quantitative studies are included. In addition, examining the "effectiveness columns" not populated by qualitative findings, might, depending on the subject nature, provide an agenda for future qualitative research. CIS, and adaptations of this method, opens new possibilities for representing a totality of evidence about a clinical topic, thus recognizing the relevance of all research literature for contributing to theories about patient care and needs.

References

Annandale E, Harvey J, Cavers D, Dixon-Woods M (2007) Gender and access to healthcare in the UK: a critical interpretive synthesis of the literature. *Evidence and Policy.* **3**(4): 463–486.

Atkins S, Lewin S, Smith H, Engel M, Fretheim A, Vomink J. (2008) Conducting a meta-ethnography of qualitative literature: Lessons learnt. *BMC Medical Research Methodology.* **8**: 21.

Brannen J (1992) *Mixing Methods: Qualitative and Quantitative Research.* Avebury, University of Michigan.

Britten N, Campbell R, Pope C, Donovan J, Morgan M, & Pill R. (2002) Using meta-ethnography to synthesise qualitative research: a worked example. *Journal of Health Services Research and Policy.* **7**(4): 209–215.

Bryman A. (1988) *Quantity and Quality in Social Research.* Unwin Hyman, London, UK pp. 5.

Campbell R, Pound P, Pope C, Britten N, Pill R, Morgan M, Donovan J. (2003) Evaluating meta-ethnography: a synthesis of qualitative research on lay experiences of diabetes and diabetes care. *Social Science and Medicine.* **56**(4): 671–684.

Coyle N. (2004) In their own words: Seven advanced cancer patients describe their experience with pain and the use of opioid drugs. *Journal of Pain and Symptom Management.* **24**: 300–309.

Dixon-Woods M, Cavers D, Agarwal S, Annandale E, Arthur A, Harvey J, Hsu R, Katbamna S, Olsen R, Smith L, Riley R, Sutton AJ. (2006) Conducting a critical interpretive synthesis of the literature on access to healthcare by vulnerable groups. *BMC Medical Research Methodology.* **6**: 35.

Dixon-Woods M, Sutton A, Shaw R, Miller T, Smith J, Young B, Bonas S, Booth A, Jones D. (2007a) Appraising qualitative research for inclusion in systematic reviews: a quantitative and qualitative comparison of three methods. *Journal of Health Services Research and Policy.* **12**(1): 42–47.

Dixon-Woods M, Booth A, Sutton AJ. (2007b) Synthesizing qualitative research: a review of published reports. *Qualitative Research.* **7**(3): 375–422.

Ersek M, Kraybill BM, Du Penn A. (1999) Factors hindering patients' use of medications for cancer pain. *Cancer Practitioner.* **7**: 226–232.

Evans D. (2002) Database searches for qualitative research. *Journal of the Medical Library Association.* **90**(3): 290–293.

Flemming K. (2007a) The knowledge base for evidence-based nursing. A role for mixed methods research? *Advances in Nursing Science.* **30**(1): 41–51.

Flemming K. (2007b) EBN Notebook: The synthesis of qualitative research and evidence-based nursing. *Evidence Based Nursing.* **10**: 68–71.

Flemming K. (2009) The use of morphine to treat cancer related pain: A synthesis of qualitative and quantitative research. *Journal of Pain and Symptom Management.* **39**(10): 139–154.

Flemming K, Briggs M. (2007) Electronic searching to locate qualitative research: evaluation of three strategies. *Journal of Advanced Nursing.* **57**(1): 95–100.

Fries CJ (2009) Bourdieu's reflexive sociology as a theoretical basis for mixed methods research: An application to complementary and alternative medicine. *Journal of Mixed Methods Research.* **3**(4): 326–348.

Greenhalgh T, Robert G, MacFarlane F, *et al.* (2005) Storylines of research in diffusion of innovation: a meta-narrative approach to systematic review. *Social Science & Medicine.* **61**: 417–430.

Guba EG, Lincoln YS (2008) Paradigmatic controversies, contradictions, and emerging confluences. In Denzin NK and Lincoln YS (eds) *The Landscape of Qualitative Research.* 3rd Edition. Sage Publications, Thousand Oaks, California.

Hammersley M (1992) *What's Wrong with Ethnography?* London, Routledge.

Hanks GW, Conno F, Cherny N, Hanna M, Kalso E, Mcquay HJ, Mercadante S, Meynadier J, Poulain P, Ripamonti C, Radbruch L, Roca I, Casas J, Sawe J, Twycross RG, Ventafridda V (2001) Morphine and alternative opioids in cancer pain: the EAPC recommendations. *British Journal of Cancer.* **84**: 587–93.

Hawker S, Payne S, Kerr C, Hardy M, Powell J. (2002) Appraising the Evidence: Reviewing disparate data systematically. *Qualitative Health Research.* **12**: 1284–1299.

Johnston-Taylor E, Ferrell BR, Grant M, Cheyney L (1993) Managing cancer pain at home: the decisions and ethical conflicts of patients, family caregivers and homecare nurses. *Oncology Nursing Forum.* **20**(6): 919–927.

Munro SA, Lewin SA, Smith HJ, Engel ME, Fretheim A, Volmink J. (2007) Patient adherence to tuberculosis treatment: A systematic review of qualitative research. *PLOS Medicine.* **4**(7): 1230–1244.

Noblit G, Hare R. (1988) *Meta-ethnography: Synthesizing Qualitative Studies.* Sage, Newbury Park, CA.

Noyes J, Popay J. (2007) Directly observed therapy and tuberculosis: how can a systematic review of qualitative research contribute to improving services? A qualitative meta-synthesis. *Journal of Advanced Nursing.* **57**(3): 227–243.

Noyes J, Popay J, Pearson A, Hannes K, Booth A. (2008) Qualitative research and Cochrane reviews. In *Cochrane Handbook for Systematic Reviews of Interventions* (Higgins J.P.T. and Green S.,eds.), Version 5.0.1, The Cochrane Collaboration, UK.

Pope C, Mays N. (2006) Synthesising qualitative research. In *Qualitative Research in Health Care* (Pope C. and Mays N., eds.), 3rd edn. Blackwell Publishing, Oxford, UK: pp. 142–52.

Reid CM, Gooberman-Hill R, Hanks GW (2008) Opioid analgesics for cancer pain: Symptom control for the living or comfort for the dying? A qualitative study to investigate the factors influencing the decision to accept morphine for pain caused by cancer. *Annals of Oncology.* **19**: 44–48.

Sale JEM, Lohfeld LH, Brazil K. (2002) Revisiting the quantitative-qualitative debate: Implications for mixed-methods research. *Quality and Quantity.* **36**, 43–53.

Sandelowski M, Barosso J. (2002) Reading qualitative studies. *International Journal of Qualitative Methods.* **1**(1): 74–108.

Schutz A. (1973) *Collected Papers Volume 1: The Problem of Social Reality.* Martinus Nijhoff, The Hague: pp. 34–47.

Sindhu DL, Dickson R. (2007) The complexity of searching the literature. *International Journal of Nursing Practice* **3**: 211–217.

Thomas J, Harden A, Oakley A, Oliver S, Sutcliffe K, Rees R, Brunton G, Kavanagh J. (2004) Integrating qualitative research with trials in systematic reviews. *BMJ.* **328**: 1010–2.

Thomas J, Harden A. (2008) Methods for the thematic synthesis of qualitative research in systematic reviews. *BMC Medical Research Methodology.* **8**: 45.

Wheeler MS. (2005) Interview with patients who have cancer and their family members. *Home Healthcare Nurse.* **23**: 642–646.

Wiffen PJ, McQuay HJ. (2007) Oral morphine for cancer pain. *Cochrane Database of Systematic Reviews*, Issue 4.

Chapter 5 The Internet in medical education: a worked example of a realist review

Geoff Wong, MD(Res)

Healthcare Innovation and Policy Unit, Centre for Health Sciences, Blizard Institute, Barts and The London School of Medicine and Dentistry, London, UK

When human agency plays an important role in producing outcomes in health service interventions, making sense of the literature base can be challenging. With human agency, individuals make decisions about whether or not to use the resources provided by the intervention in question under the influence of the context in which they and the intervention is situated. This produces non-linear or semi- (demi-) regular patterns of behavior that ultimately "produce" (or not) the desired outcome(s). Any review method that is going to make sense of such interventions needs to have some means of taking account of the influence of context on human decision-making. Furthermore, it needs to be able to provide generalizable explanations of why certain interventions work and also the circumstances in which they will work. It is from these generalizable explanations that lessons can be learnt about how best in the future to design and implement similar interventions. One review method that has been developed specifically for, and rises up to, the challenges of making sense of human agency mediated interventions is realist review. In this chapter, a "walk-through" of the realist review method is provided using the example of a review of the use of the Internet in medical education.

Introduction

A realist review (or synthesis – the terms are synonymous) is a type of theory-driven qualitative systematic review method that has been developed by Pawson to enable reviewers to synthesize evidence from seemingly heterogeneous interventions (Pawson 2006). Realist reviews center on the interplay between human agency and context and are an evolution of the work done by Pawson and Tilley on realist evaluations (Pawson & Tilley 1997). Their main

Synthesizing Qualitative Research: Choosing the Right Approach, First Edition.
Edited by Karin Hannes and Craig Lockwood.
© 2012 John Wiley & Sons, Ltd. Published 2012 by John Wiley & Sons, Ltd.

goal is not so much to prove that an intervention works, but more to explain "how," "why," "for whom," "in what circumstances," and "to what extent" it works. It is thus more about generating understanding about interventions and from this understanding enabling causal inferences to be made about how they might best be made to work in the future. The main uses for realist reviews are either to help review teams provide recommendations about interventions to decision- or policymakers and/or to assist researchers in designing "better" interventions and/or directing their research efforts.

In this chapter I will first introduce the theoretical underpinnings of realist reviews (Part 1) and then move on to provide an outline of the review process as well as examples of the theory in action later on (in Part 2).

PART 1: PRINCIPLES

In the health sciences, realist review has and is being used to better understand what are often called complex interventions (Greenhalgh *et al.* 2007; Shepperd *et al.* 2009). A number of definitions or descriptions exist as to the exact nature of complex interventions, but for the purposes of this chapter I would suggest complex interventions may best be understood as human agency-mediated interventions and that the definition in Box 5.1 best describes their pertinent features.

The main rationale for the use of this review method lies in the "fit" between the theoretical assumptions and principles which underlie both realist review and complex interventions. Much of what follows in this section is drawn from the seminal work by Pawson in his 2006 book *Evidence-based Policy. A Realist Perspective* (2006).

Box 5.1 A definition of complex interventions (adapted from Craig *et al.* 2008 and Anderson 2008)

Complex interventions consist of:
- Multiple components that make up the intervention.
- Components consists mainly (but not exclusively) of humans and the resources provided by the intervention.
- It is the interactions between the components that produce the intervention's outcomes.
- Human decision-making influences the nature of these interactions.
- The various components of the intervention do not interact in a linear and deterministic way with each other.
- The interactions are influenced by the context within and beyond the intervention.

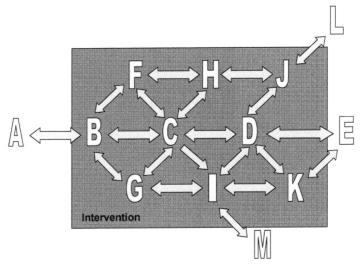

Figure 5.1 A highly simplified diagram to illustrate some of the possible components of a complex intervention.

In complex interventions, human beings (be they, for example, the researchers, the participants, or any individual involved in the intervention) often make up many of the components that interact within certain contexts to generate outcomes. The other set of components that will be relevant might (for example) be the resources that are made available to those involved in the intervention. The human "components" make choices about the use (or not) of the resources provided as part of the intervention during its implementation. It is the accumulation of the choices that have been made at each decision point that produces (or not) the final outcome(s) (Figure 5.1). Pawson has pointed out that in complex interventions there often exists a chain of events (which he terms the "program theory") of varying lengths through which the intervention "causes" its final outcome. Thus, if we look within the "black box" of a complex intervention, we see a myriad of possible pathways that the human "components" may take, but only some will generate the desired outcome(s) of the intervention. Whilst there are myriad potential paths through a complex intervention, the contexts that are associated (at every level) with and beyond the intervention have a significant influence on which pathways are more likely to be taken.

Importantly, the choices that are available to these human "components" are not infinite, but are influenced and to an extent dictated by the context in which they find themselves. Thus the context in which a complex

Context + Mechanism = Outcome

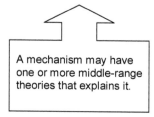

Figure 5.2 Explaining the relationship between context, mechanism, and outcome.

intervention takes place will have some degree of influence on the outcomes of such an intervention by "limiting" the choices that the human "components" can make. This interplay between context, choice making and outcomes has been encapsulated by Pawson and Tilley (Pawson 2006; Pawson & Tilley 1997) in the "equation" $C + M = O$ where C is Context, M is Mechanism and O is outcome (Figure 5.2). The context influences which mechanism(s) will "fire" in order to produce outcome(s). Within the realm of health services research, a mechanism can best be thought of as people making decisions about the resources presented before them. Mechanisms are thus "things which go on" within an individual's head that then goes on to produce an outcome (or outcomes). Within any mechanism there may exist further mechanisms.

The involvement of humans in complex interventions introduces the element of non-linear causality. Humans do not always make the same choices each and every time. However, because their choices are influenced by the context they find themselves in, under certain contexts some choices are more likely to occur than others. So whilst it would be impossible to always predict what choices a person might make, the influence of context is such that semi-predictable patterns of "choice making" occurs under certain contexts – something termed demi-regularities (or demi-regs) by Pawson (2003). Within a realist review, because the review team is analyzing reported data, the demi-regularities manifest themselves as semi-predictable patterns in the data.

One of the key tasks of realist reviews is the identification of these demi-regularities and importantly to explain the how, why, in what circumstances, for whom, and to what extent about them. Demi-regularities are the result of context firing mechanism(s) to produce outcomes. If a demi-regularity is noted across a set of interventions, then the same mechanism may well be present, but it may be "fired" to differing degrees in each intervention because

Box 5.2 Definitions of theory and middle-range theory (4)

Theory:
There are multiple definitions for theory but for the purposes of this chapter, "A theory is an attempt to organize the facts – some 'proven', some more conjectural – within a domain of inquiry into a structurally coherent system." (Klee 1997)

Middle-range theory:
This is a theory that lies "...between the minor but necessary working hypotheses that evolve in abundance during day-to-day research and the all-inclusive systematic efforts to develop a unified theory that will explain all the observed uniformities of social behavior, social organization and social change...

It is intermediate to general theories of social systems which are too remote from particular classes of social behavior, organization and change to account for what is observed and to those detailed orderly descriptions of particulars that are not generalized at all. *Middle-range theory involves abstraction, of course, but they are close enough to observed data to be incorporated in propositions that permit empirical testing.*[my emphases]" (Merton 1967)

of the contextual differences. It is these context-influenced demi-regular patterns of choice-making about resources that allows for generalizability across complex interventions. Importantly, why certain decisions are made within certain contexts can be explained and understood through the use of middle-range theory (or theories) (see Box 5.2 for definitions of theory and middle-range theory). The middle-range theories attempt to explain the mechanisms that are fired in the demi-regularities and may be novel (derived by the review team) or (more likely) have been described previously by other researchers.

The central concepts in realist review are based on the various sociological theories of human agency that have been developed over the last century.[1] Human agency and its relationships to societal structures has been and still is hotly contested in sociology. Amongst the theorists that support human agency, there is general consensus that humans tend to make certain choices under certain circumstances (contexts) that changes the position they are in within the world they exist in. In turn, this "changed" world then further influences the decisionmaker. Thus what consensus there is argues for the importance of context in human decision-making (Adams & Sydie 2001).

---

[1] The various sociological theories that realist review has drawn upon and the debates that surround them is beyond the scope of this chapter. Readers who are interested in this topic are directed to Adams and Sydie's *Sociological Theory* (reference 11 below).

What Pawson has done is to weave together and develop the numerous theories of how and why certain outcomes occur as a result of human decision-making, under certain contexts, into a review method. Furthermore, he has highlighted that the demi-regularities and their associated mechanisms that can be indentified within complex interventions form the key to making sense of the heterogeneous data that is invariably found within such interventions. It is then through middle-range theories that these demi-regularities and their associated mechanisms may be explained and allow for inferences to be made about what might happen when seemingly similar complex interventions are implemented in the future. Finally, though (as we shall see in the next section) realist review has a series of stages and processes, it is best though of as, "...a set of principles intended to inspire a particular approach rather than to spell out a set of techniques. Each inquiry has to grapple with a different set of contexts, mechanisms and outcomes and thus specific techniques need to be brought on board 'as appropriate'." (R Pawson. Personal communication, 2009).

PART 2: REALIST REVIEW – A WORKED EXAMPLE

In the remainder of this chapter, I will outline the stages in a realist review and illustrate how each stage may be operationalized with examples and findings from a realist review in medical education in which I was the lead reviewer of the review team. I will explain the thinking behind the decisions we made as a review team and also highlight some of the challenges a realist reviewer faces whilst undertaking a realist review. I will also provide illustrative examples of how the theory and principles behind realist review can be seen in action in our review. Finally, it is worth pointing out that though the example I have provided is drawn from medical education, I have deliberately attempted to draw out the processes, lessons, and recommendations from this example which are applicable in reviewing complex interventions in any field.

Internet-based medical education: a realist review of what works, for whom, and in what circumstances

An important initial decision point is whether or not the realist review method is appropriate. A realist review should ideally be undertaken when the outcome(s) of interest in an intervention is likely to be the result of human agency under contextual influences and when the goal of the review is sense-making and not judgment. This does not mean that all of the chain of events has to involve human agency, but that you suspect that there is a good chance that in trying to answer your review question(s), human agency does have an influence on the outcomes found in the body of literature you intend to review.

We began our review in 2006 and it represents the first ever use of the realist review method in medical education. The review was completed in 2008 and is freely available online (http://www.biomedcentral.com/1472-6920/10/12 [accessed 7 June 2011]) (Wong *et al.* 2010) Our rationale for using the realist review method was that we believed that medical educational interventions which use the Internet to teach are complex interventions. Within this form of education, our observation (from the literature and as tutors on an Internet-based course) was that learners often had to make choices about whether or not to use and learn from the resources provided to them by an Internet-based course (see Box 5.3 as an example).

Box 5.3   An example of the components, context, and middle-range theory in a complex intervention

A common type of Internet based resource used is the electronic textbook (where text and often multimedia is made available online). Jao *et al.* offered just such a resource with the goal of increasing medical students' knowledge of neurology on a compulsory placement (Jao *et al.* 2005). They provided a free electronic neurology textbook and based all their teaching and end of placement assessments exclusively on the contents of their electronic textbook. They reported that students' knowledge of neurology increased and the electronic textbook was well received and used. In contrast many other interventions using electronic textbooks do not achieve their set goal(s).

To understand the apparent "success" of this intervention the realist reviewer needs to identify the various components, their interactions, and the theories that might explain the outcomes reported.

In this example the medical students are the ones who make the decisions. The resource is the electronic textbook and the context consists of things like, it is a neurology placement, the compulsory nature of the neurology placement, the placement's assessment process, and any alternative "competing" learning resources available (such as the face-to-face teaching provided). The placement also had tutors and fellows students and they represent the other components of the intervention with whom interaction can take place.

In this one example a series of steps (which may occur in series and/or in parallel) needs to take place before a medical student might learn any neurology on this neurology placement. The review team's task is to identify any demi-regularities and their corresponding mechanisms and then test their candidate middle-range theory (or theories). The purpose of this process being to explain in this one intervention (or course) why the students used (or did not use) the electronic textbook and how its use resulted in an increase in knowledge.

The realist review process

In realist review an outline protocol is first developed, and Pawson *et al.* have broken down the realist review process into a series of stages (Figure 5.3) (Pawson *et al.* 2005). However, it must be borne in mind that this has only been done for sake of clarity. In fact, a realist review team must be prepared to; (a) run some stages in parallel; (b) iteratively modify their initial protocol and; (c) revisit (if necessary) every stage of the review process as the review progresses. Thus, in reality, the review process is not linear but iterative (as illustrated in Figure 5.3) and each of the stages outlined in a realist review may be not only running in parallel, but also revisited or refined as a review progresses and new demi-regularities, mechanisms, and/or middle-range theories are encountered and need to be "tested" against the manuscripts included in a review. However, we suggest that each change should be documented for the sake of transparency.

Stage 1: defining the scope of the review

This stage of the review is necessarily very exploratory and fluid since what is done will very much depend on not only what the research question and purpose of the review is but also what is found during the review.

Identification of the research question

As with all research, a realist review must begin with an initial research question. The question may be very broad to start off with as the review team might be unsure as to whether or not the data exists to answer their question. Then, as the review progresses, it may be that the review team has to progressively narrow their review question based on their emerging findings. Development of the research question should ideally take into account the views of those who will ultimately wish to use the results of the review or outstanding research priorities.

In our review, the family of seemingly similar complex interventions we chose to look at was the use of the Internet to teach doctors. Our initial research question was: "*What is it about the Internet that works in medical education, for whom, in what circumstances, in what respect and why?*". We started out with such a broad question because though we were familiar with the literature, we were still unsure if there was sufficient detail contained within the literature to address our question in full. As I have already mentioned, no previous realist review had been undertaken in this field. While we had the methodological expertise (in Professor Pawson) to know what type of data was needed, it was not until we had formally and systematically searched the literature that were we aware of its nature.

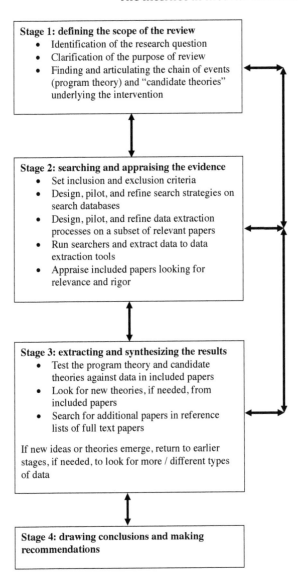

Figure 5.3 Diagram showing the stages and iterative nature of realist reviews.

As you will see later on, we encountered a series of issues around our included studies that made us narrow down our ambitions. In summary, the detail reported in our included studies only allowed us to identify and explain certain sections of the chain of events (or program theory).

On the point of utility to users of your review, as we worked and researched in the field of medical education we were quite familiar with the issues around the research and literature in this field. What we knew was that educators increasingly wanted to know more about the situations when Internet-based education should be used, as opposed to if it worked better compared to other teaching methods. This shift in discourse on Internet-based teaching seemed to us to be something that was potentially answerable through realist review.

Clarification of the purpose of the review

Our review initially had two purposes; 1) to address the review question (see above) and; 2) as a methodological enquiry into the use of realist review in a field where it had not been used before. As mentioned above, we knew that the "burning" question in the use of the Internet in medical education was to understand more about the contexts of when it should be used. We felt that our funding permitted us to explore this "need" (i.e. the "for whom," "to what extent," and "in what circumstances"). We felt that the most useful set of findings we could come up with were; 1) a chain of events (or program theory) that could be applied across the whole family of Internet interventions rather than focusing in too much detail on any one specific type of use of the Internet; and 2) identification of mechanisms and their associated middle-range theory (or theories) that were generalizable. We also hoped that, as we ran this review, we would learn lessons about its utility in the field of medical education.

Time and resources are always a constraint on how much of an initially broad research question a review team can answer. Hence a useful "survival" step is to expect that a realist review can only be expected to take a particular "cut," focus, or emphasis through the research literature, but more "cuts" could be taken depending on the time available for the review. For example, a synthesis might only focus on "why" and "how" but not have time or resources to discover more about the "for whom," "in what circumstances," and "in what respect" and "to what extent." Another way to "cut" the literature may be to focus on specific contexts (e.g. only community based interventions) or narrower intervention types (e.g. only weight loss programs in diabetics). The risk is of course to the generalizability of the findings, but it may be that even taking this narrower cut, a review team uncovers a mechanism that also operates more broadly (e.g. a mechanism that operates in weight loss programs for diabetics also operates in all weight loss programs). If a review team suspects this, time permitting, they might be able to test this middle-range theory in intervention types where they suspect that the same mechanism might be present.

Finding and articulating the chain of events (program theory)
and "candidate theories" underlying the intervention

It may or not be possible at this stage for the review team to start to construct an initial chain of events (or program theory) that explains the steps required to bring about the desired outcome(s) in the complex interventions of interest. This initial "exploratory" chain does not have to be correct, but acts as a starting point in the review team's journey to understanding what the "active ingredients" are in any family of seemingly similar complex intervention and/ or in interventions where they think similar mechanisms might be operation. Thus this initial chain should be a representation of how, on the whole, "things happen" for the complex interventions of interest. A useful analogy is to think of this step as being about looking inside the "black box" of the interventions of interest and seeing what is inside and how the contents all fit together. It is very likely that once the review team has started to sift through the evidence, they will modify their chain accordingly. Determining what the chain may look like is initially a mixture of guess work and the review team's knowledge of the field and literature. We found that brain-storming and discussion of the possible pathways amongst the review team was a useful starting point.

However, it may be that what the chain does consist of is less clear at this point. This is fine, as during the review process the review team is likely to gain some insight into the complex intervention of interest and thus be able to "fill in the blanks" as the review progresses. This was the position we found ourselves in both at the beginning and end of our review! We realized that within the chain there must have been some "things that occurred" that enabled students to learn (i.e. that learning was a mechanism that needed "unpacking"), but what these consisted of and how they fitted together was unclear at the outset. We also realized (as our review progressed) that getting students to engage with the learning was a key mechanism, but how this tied into the learning and what explained why some students might engage and other not was less clear. Thus our initial chain consisted of only two obvious mechanisms (learning and engagement) and thus was rather sketchy – "filling in the blanks" was one of our key priorities.

Whether or not a review team has a clear chain in mind, it is still important to try to address the question as to what mechanisms and their associated middle-range theories they think may be in operation in the complex interventions of interest. Pawson has called these "candidate [middle-range] theories" and the "search" for these will need to be flexible, iterative, and intuitive. Fortunately for us, in medical education a large literature base on the theoretical aspects of education already existed and therefore we thought that for theories on "learning" and possibly even engaging students, it was unlikely that we would need to "re-invent the wheel." However, a review team's field of interest and expertise may be different and so unfortunately there is no simple formula for this phase of a realist review. Our experience was that personal knowledge of the literature, specialist library collections, discussion with peers and experts in the field and within the review team were reasonable starting points.

Selecting which theories to follow further and which to discard is not an easy process and requires a degree of subjective judgment. We made our decisions based on: whether or not the theory or framework was likely to answer our review's research question; focusing on (what we thought were) the most generalizable mechanisms initially and; assessing how ubiquitous (e.g. cited) a theory, model, or framework was.

Review teams should at this point consider what sort of data might be needed from research studies in order to answer the research question(s) and to begin the creation of data extraction "template(s)" that is/are able to capture the relevant data. For example, in our review, we knew that we would need to gather both qualitative (e.g. to answer the "how" and "why" questions) and some quantitative data (e.g. for the "for whom" question) – in Stage 3 (below) we explain what we did and why.

Challenges

As a final note to this stage it is worth pointing out that this is the "hardest" part of a realist review and has been called the "swamp" by Trisha Greenhalgh (Pawson *et al.* 2005). It is hard because the temptation is to try to ask a realist review to do too much. If the outcome(s) of a complex intervention are partly the results of human agency and there might be a long chain of events (or program theory) involved, then there are likely to be a plethora of potentially fruitful areas that may need closer scrutiny and examination during a realist review. Time and resources are the main initial constraints and so deciding on what particular aspect to focus on (and what to leave out) and how to construct a chain, as well as which candidate theories to start with, all become pressing and seemingly insoluble questions.

We would want to reassure potential review teams that the "swamp" is not endless. We found that a number of important strategies assisted us. These included:

- Focusing a review on the pressing questions in a field of research. What do fellow researchers, clinicians, patients, or policy and decisionmakers want answers to?
- A review team should do its best in constructing a chain of events (or program theory). It does not matter if it is initially "wrong" as the whole point of the review is to try to uncover what it does consist of and a review team is likely to only be able to fully clarify it once they have looked in the

literature. It may even be that at the end of a review, a review team is only able to uncover some parts of a chain.

- Review teams should have to decide which middle-range theories may be in operation in a chain. Many theories on how or why things "work" abound, often in other disciplines, so review teams should cast their nets widely in their initial search for candidate theories. It may be that in your field of interest there are too many competing theories. If this is the case then rather than agonise over exactly which ones are more correct and hence need to be tested first, try one of the following: a) go for the most popular; b) focus on the theories that are most likely to address your research question and/or the needs of your "users;" and/or c) have an educated guess. Again, it does not matter if the initial "guesses" were wrong. Realist reviews are about uncovering and testing middle-range theories.

Finally, remember that realist reviews are iterative. The initial "protocol" is not set in stone, but is meant to be modified in light of the findings and increased understanding of the complex intervention of interest. Review teams should make sure that they document and justify the changes they made in their review process and outcomes of any decisions made for transparency's sake.

Stage 2: searching for and appraising the evidence
Searching for the evidence
In this stage, the purpose of searching is to identify from the literature a body of evidence from which the review team may elucidate a chain of events (or program theory) and test candidate theories.

Deciding and defining the sampling strategy, sources, and methods used
The goal in realist synthesis is not necessarily to seek out every relevant article in the field of enquiry, but to obtain a representative "maximum variety sample" against which to test the candidate theories. We have found that this type of sample is most informative because it contains both examples of "successful" and "unsuccessful" interventions. Such examples from both ends of the spectrum tended to allow us to gain greater insights and understanding as to the important aspects of a complex intervention that might have made it "work" or not – something often called "flows" and "barriers" to success by Pawson.

What this sample will consist of and where to look for it will depend initially on the focus of the research question and topic. Many of the familiar search techniques regularly used in systematic reviews are applicable in searching out such a sample and the strategies and sources used in previous reviews are a good start (Haig & Dozier 2003a, b). We found that in order to obtain a maximum variety sample, we set very broad inclusion criteria and looked in a large number of databases (for more details of our search strategy and terms, please refer to Additional File 1 of our published report – see above for link). As you will see later, realist review does not have a hierarchy of evidence, and data to test theory may come from a variety of research designs. Hence study designs of any kind were included in our review as long as they: had medical doctors (at any training stage) as participants; somehow used the Internet for teaching; and had some form of evaluation data.

However, in a realist review, review teams have to be prepared to re-run searches or return to excluded articles, when (for example) data emerges that requires new candidate theories to be sought out or tested. The searching process is thus not only iterative, but also guided by the need to keep searching for and testing middle-range theories that are best able to account for the demi-regularities encountered. Because of this need to keep seeking data to test middle-range theories we found that more directed search strategies, like snowballing, personal contacts, or asking experts in the field, were more productive (Greenhalgh & Peacock 2005).

On a practical note, use of some sort of citation tracking software is a good idea, as is making sure search histories are saved. The former allows review teams to keep track of not only what they have found, but also to "file" a list of the references they have used and not used to test your middle-range theories on. Knowing where references have been "filed" is important due to the iterative nature of the review process – as review teams never know when they might need to turn to an article they had earlier discarded as seemingly irrelevant! The function of the latter will mean that review teams do not have to always start from scratch every time they need to search for literature with a slightly different focus.

This is probably the aspect of the realist review process that is most familiar to secondary researchers and so many of the searching skills learnt in other review methods will be applicable.

Setting the threshold for stopping searching at saturation

Realist review uses the concept of saturation to guide when it would be reasonable to stop searching for data from further articles on which to test the candidate middle-range theories (Pawson 2006). When to stop will always be a matter of judgment for the review team but any decision must be clearly justified and documented. Whilst we did not stop at saturation in our review as we wanted to explore the validity of this process in our review, we would recommend that review teams adhere to this convention. Instead we extracted and synthesized data for theory testing from all the 249 separate articles that were found in our search of 15 different electronic databases.

From our review, it was hard to judge if stopping at saturation would have helped or hindered the review. One advantage we noted from not stopping at saturation was that we able to identify a number of different families of contexts which proved to be exemplar examples with which to test our middle-range theories. We had no way of knowing in advance that this would be the case as only after going through all 249 articles did this become clear.

Appraising the evidence

In a realist review, an entire study is rarely the appropriate unit of analysis. Furthermore, a distinction needs to be made about data that has been used to build theory and to test theory. For the former, so called "quality" and rigor is likely to be much less important. Within any one included article, a reviewer may only find particular pieces of data of use in theory testing. It is therefore appropriate that studies are not included or excluded on a single judgment about their quality, but are done so on what relevance they bring and how rigorously they have been conducted (Box 5.4). Studies are selected not just on methodological quality but also on overall fitness for purpose (e.g. what can this study tell me about the causal chain and my candidate theories?). In terms of rigor, the decision needs to be made at the point of when the data is being considered for use and then judgments can be made about how plausible that piece of data is rather than the study in its entirety. In our review, we did not encounter a single included article where we noted that the segments of data we needed from it were insufficiently rigorous so as to constitute grounds for rejection.

Box 5.4 Definitions of relevance and rigor in realist reviews (adapted from Pawson 2006)

Relevance – in realist review is not about whether a study covers a particular topic, but more if it helps to support or refute the candidate theory under scrutiny (i.e., can it make a contribution?)

Rigor – if a particular inference is drawn by the original researcher has it sufficient weight to make a methodologically credible contribution to test a particular candidate theory (i.e., what sort of a contribution does it make?)? When considering rigor, this is where judgment needs to be exercised by the reviewers as to the methodological quality of the study. However, the judgment of the rigor of a trial is not a "black and white" one where a whole study is rejected based on its performance against a rating scale of some sort. It is more about appreciating that most studies have strengths and weaknesses and that some of a study's findings may well have come from sections of the study that were methodologically sound, but others from where it was not.

Challenges

The main challenge in this stage of a realist review is in finding enough of the "right" kind of data with which to test candidate theories. We have found that an advantage of realist reviews is that there is no bar to the type of study design from which theory-testing data might be drawn. While this may "broaden the field" of included studies, we have three tips that review teams may wish to consider:

- Within any included paper, we suggest that you scour all sections of the paper in your search for theory-testing data. Our experience is that nuggets of useful information may be found in any section of included papers.
- Be prepared to search not just in the databases usually suggested by researchers in the field, but also in those that are closely related or that might (in the review team's judgment) be relevant. For example, in our review, though we were looking at medical education, we decided to also search in purely educational databases (e.g. Education Resource Information Center, British Education Index, British Education Internet Resource Catalogue, Education on-line, and Research and Development Resource Base).
- Do be curious. If an included paper mentions or suggests a theory or idea that might seem relevant, do find the time to pursue it or at the very least check that it is not. We found that this might be done quite quickly by just scanning abstracts or through a "quick and dirty" search on an Internet search engine. Our experience is that useful middle-range theories often come from other disciplines and one of the ways to access these disciplines is to combine curiosity with directed searching.

Stage 3: extracting and synthesizing the results

In realist reviews, data extraction and synthesis are closely intertwined processes that run in parallel, but I have deliberately and artificially separated them in order to be able to explain each in detail.

Extracting the data

The type of data that needs to be extracted for theory testing will be determined by the research question and influenced by initial ideas on the possible chain of events (or program theory) and candidate theories. The purpose of the data extraction is to allow the review team to capture important aspects of the included articles to assist the synthesis process. It can best be seen as a collection and documentation process that sets the stage for synthesis. In effect the review team is trying to gather into a manageable and searchable "pile" all the pieces of information scoured from the included papers that will aid the synthesis process.

The "template" used will have been developed (e.g., at Stage 1), refined (through piloting – for example on a subset of relevant articles) as a review progresses. In our review we extracted descriptive information about our included studies along with our interpretation of how and/or why a study contributed to theory testing, into Microsoft's Excel spreadsheet (see Box 5.5 for details of the type of data we extracted to our spreadsheet). We found that as we had so many papers to extract data from (249 in total) we needed a way of summarizing the pertinent aspects of each included paper so that we could quickly and easily refer to it during data synthesis.

Box 5.5 Details of the type of data we extracted from included studies to our Excel spreadsheet

- Document name (as identified in referencing software)
- Author(s)
- Publication year
- Language
- Country of study
- Source (name of journal)
- Full reference
- Study aim(s)
- Number of subjects
- Age range
- Gender (mix)
- Professional mix
- Topic area
- Educational setting
- Interaction (level)
- Technological context (e.g. type of Internet connection available)
- Cost/access
- How was the Internet used
- Description of study design
- Validity/reliability of instruments/study
- Findings (e.g. positive/negative/mixed)
- Outcome measures
- Educational consequences
- Educational alternative
- Summary of results
- How and Why?
- For whom?
- To what extent?
- In what circumstances?
- Change theories based on study?
- What is the paper trying to show?
- Competing interests
- Notes

As we synthesized our data, we added additional sections ("columns") to our spreadsheet in an attempt to provide a richer summary description and overview of our included studies. This iterative process also entailed us re-reading papers that we had already extracted data from in order to ensure that our spreadsheet was consistently populated. To further assist the synthesis process we used the qualitative research software NVivo (2002) to code sections of texts that we thought might be useful in theory testing. We used NVivo mainly as a "searchable filing system" as we had a large number of included papers in our review. One advantage we found in its use was that it made it very easy for us to extract the verbatim text from our included papers for various purposes (e.g., during team discussions, for writing and publication, etc.)

When using NVivo, we coded sections of text in our included papers based on both inductively and deductively derived codes. So, for example, we coded inductively for issues that were mentioned repeatedly, with the goal that we might later (in the synthesis step – see below) be able to account for these through a middle-range theory. Our deductive codes came from our can-didate theories, so, for example, we had codes for "interaction" and "feedback" which were derived from Laurillard's Conversational Framework (Laurillard 2002) (see below for more details).

Synthesizing the findings

Data synthesis should start the moment data is being extracted. Data extraction provides the "raw" data and one of the review team's first tasks is to try to identify any demi-regularities that may be present in the data from their included studies. Then the review team's task turns to trying to make some sense of the relationship between their initial chain of events (or program theory), mechanisms, and candidate (middle-range) theories and the demi-regularities they have identified. The overall goal at this stage is to address the question, "*Is our initial understanding of the complex intervention supported by what we have found in our included studies? If not, why not and how do we need to change our understanding?*" This understanding should be questioned on a number of levels; a) is the chain of event (or program theory) correctly described or does it need to be modified?; and b) have we identified the appropriate middle-range theory (or theories) that is/are able to explain the influences of context on the mechanism(s) that are operating in the chain of events (or program theory)?

Data synthesis follows similar principles to those found more generally in qualitative research. At its core is interpretation and the key processes employed are immersion (reading and re-reading of included papers), discussion amongst members of the review team, and repeated theory

> **Box 5.6** Some key questions to use when testing candidate theories
>
> - How does this article add to my understanding of the research question, if at all?
> - Which, if any, of the candidate theories does the data in this article refer to?
> - How does what I have found compare and contrast to the findings from different studies?
> - Have I found findings that are both confirmatory and contradictory?
> - Do I need to refine my candidate theories in light of the evidence?
> - Could another theory explain what I have found?

testing. When interpreting the data, we drew on the texts within our included articles, our Excel spreadsheet, and NVivo codes to try to identify prominent demi-regularities and the contexts in which they operated. We then tested our initial candidate middle-range theories by seeing if they were able to explain why these demi-regularities occurred under the contexts reported in our included papers using a series of questions (Box 5.6). If a candidate theory was not able to do so then we sought new candidates. Thus each candidate theory was repeatedly subjected to testing as we worked our way through our maximum variety sample of included articles.

Importantly when we identified what might prove to be an important demi-regularity or candidate theory, we revisited the included articles we had extracted data from earlier in our review in order to seek out the presence of the "new" demi-regularity or test the "new" candidate theory.

The final "product" of any realist synthesis is an answer to the initial research question that uses "successful" middle-range theories to explain the mechanisms that are present in a chain of events (or program theory). A middle-range theory can be considered to be "successful" when it is able to explain (for example) how and why certain patterns of outcomes are likely to occur under certain contexts – that is, it can explain the demi-regularities.

Laurillard's Conversational Framework and Rogers Diffusion of Innovations

In our review we started out with four candidate theories: Laurillard's Conversational Framework (CF) (Laurillard 2002), Schon's reflective practitioner (Schon 1987), Slotnick's 'How doctors learn' (Slotnick 1996), and Reeves' 'Effective dimensions of interactive learning' (Reeves 2005). By the end of our review we had discarded three and added an additional one, leaving us with Laurillard's Conversational Framework (CF) and Rogers Diffusion of Innovation (Innovation theory) (Rogers 1995).

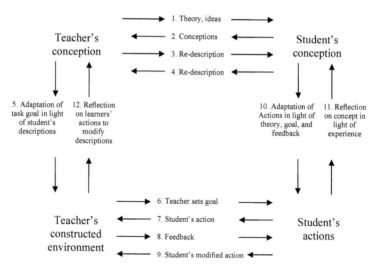

Figure 5.4 A diagrammatic representation of Laurillard's Conversational Framework.

As we progressed with data extraction and synthesis, we found that the CF (Figure 5.4) was able to explain a prominent demi-regularity that we had noted in our included papers – that is the constant reference to "interaction" being important in Internet-based courses. To be more specific we noted that in Internet-based courses that were "interactive" learners were more likely to rate them more highly and have greater knowledge gains compared to non/less "interactive" courses.

In brief, the CF is built on the theory that a learner learns by entering into a dialog with others (virtual or human) in order to clarify understanding and obtain feedback on their understanding and/or performance. Examples of the type of verbatim texts we used to support the CF can be found in Box 5.7. The "interaction" demi-regularity could thus be understood in terms of learners' wish for more dialog and feedback as a way of learning when using Internet-based courses. While there is without doubt more to our "learning" mechanism, we had begun to gain a better understanding of it through the CF and its explanation of the "interaction" demi-regularity.

It was only after we had begun our review that we noted that learner engagement might be an important mechanism. This proved to be the case as we found that in many of our included studies use of the Internet-based resource on offer had patchy uptake. None of our initial candidate theories were able to explain learner engagement. However, as we continued to extract and synthesize data from our included studies, we noted a comment in one article that suggested that Internet-based interventions might best be

Box 5.7 Examples of verbatim text used to support the CF

"The interactive dialog probably played a large role in the program's effective-ness by encouraging the students to work through problems, inducing them to take more time on particular tasks and probably to give more attention to the material." (Grundman *et al.* 2000)

"When asked to design an effective learning tool for this e-course, the students unanimously said they wanted interactivity—interactive quizzes and interactive cases.... Students want e-courses to be built around cases, quizzes, and con-versations with teachers." (Hoban *et al.* 2003)

"After surveying the students, the modular and dynamic teaching approach of simPHYSIO (interactivity, user driven manipulations, animations) was one of the most significant features in helping the student learn the material and enjoy the learning process..." "I like the interactive approach of virtual labs. It made the concepts easier to understand." (Huang 2003)

understood as innovations. This finding was discussed amongst our review team and when we started to use the "lens" of innovation to interpret our extracted data – through an adaptation of Rogers' Diffusion of Innovation Theory (Table 5.1), we found that this lens helped us to make more sense of some of our raw data.

Three prominent demi-regularities within engagement emerged from our included papers. First, we noted that learners continually looked for reasons

Table 5.1 Diffusion of innovations theory and its attributes

Attributes (adapted from Rogers 1995 and Moore and Benbasat 1991)

Compatibility: Innovations that are compatible with the values, norms, and perceived needs of intended adopters will be more easily adopted and implemented.
Ease of use (complexity): Innovations that are perceived by key players as simple to use will be more easily adopted and implemented.
Relative advantage: Innovations that have a clear, unambiguous advantage in terms of either effectiveness or cost-effectiveness will be more easily adopted and implemented. If a potential user sees no relative advantage in the innovation he or she does not generally consider it further: in other words, relative advantage is a *sine qua non* for adoption. Relative advantage is a socially constructed phenomenon.
Trialabililty: Innovations that can be experimented with by intended users on a limited basis will be more easily adopted and implemented.
Observability: If the benefits of an innovation are visible to intended adopters, it will be more easily adopted and implemented.
Re-invention: If a potential adopter can adapt, refine, or otherwise modify the innovation to suit his or her own needs, it will be more easily adopted and implemented.

as to why they should bother to use any Internet-based resource that was offered to them. This could be directly mapped onto the "relative advantage" (or perceived usefulness) attribute of Rogers' theory (Table 5.1). Second, learners were more likely to engage with Internet-based resources that were easy to use – an observation which mapped onto the "ease of use" attribute. Finally, the use of the Internet resource had to align with the value and norms of learners if it were to stand any chance of being used – an observation that mapped onto the "compatibility" attribute. We further identified that there were specific recurrent contexts which consistently influenced the "relative advantage" attribute. These were: access to learning; access to consistent content; links with assessment; convenience; cost saving; interactivity; and time saving. On a methodological point, within a realist review Rogers' attributes would be considered sub-mechanism within the "over arching" engagement mechanism.

What we then did was to re-read our included articles (from the start) to look for more evidence of the aforementioned behaviors in order test Rogers' Innovation Theory and its three attributes – "compatibility," "ease of use," and "relative advantage." Examples of the type of verbatim texts we used to support the Innovation Theory can be found in Box 5.8.

Box 5.8 Examples of verbatim text used to support some of the attributes of the Diffusion of Innovations Theory

"The advantages for group work were repeatedly mentioned (28 respondents), with comments including: 'Great because everyone sees the same image and people aren't staring down a microscope — so are more able to talk', 'I enjoyed it because you and your partner were looking at the same slide so it was easier to talk about it', 'Virtual slides provide a very clear image, easier to use and to discuss. Easier to ask questions and good for interactive learning.'"(Kumar et al. 2004)

"Nevertheless, the preceptors felt that this type of presentation allowed better use of limited resources. It enabled them to reach a broader audience with nominal extra time. They felt that it was most beneficial to the site B (distant teaching site) residents, who may experience more difficulties accessing these teaching sessions." (Kroeker et al. 2000)

"We have concluded that while [Internet-mediated] videoconferencing provides many advantages over both telephone conferencing and regional conference programmes, it still remains inferior in terms of acceptability to CME consumers compared with our existing regional conference programmes. This is largely because the consumers felt that they lacked the interpersonal contact in videoconferencing. However, most did admit that they would use videoconferencing if the regional conference programme were withdrawn and they certainly found it superior to telephone conferencing."(Davis & McCracken 2002)

Challenges

Data

We found that it was not possible for us to find sufficient fine-grain detail in our included studies to test each and every stage in the CF nor all the attributes of the Innovations Theory. The detail of the reporting in our included studies was such that only an overall "broad brush" need for dialog and feedback could be supported (and not refuted) and we found no data to support the attributes of "trialability," "observability," and "reinvention." We had hoped that by having very broad and permissive inclusion criteria we could avoid this issue of "missing data," but the paucity of reporting educational context and theory is a well recognized problem in medical education and we were unable to overcome this issue. How pervasive and prominent this problem is will depend on your topic area. What we found was that certain search techniques were helpful in "filling in the blanks" for each included article where more detailed data was needed to permit theory testing. These included: checking the reference lists of full text articles for further studies; searching under specific authors in databases or online; and looking for more "grey" literature – such as reports, theses, or conference papers. The implications of this limitation are discussed in Stage 4 below.

Rigor

An issue that deserves attention at this point is the use of multiple reviewers in the searching, appraising, extraction, and synthesis stages of realist reviews. What has to be borne in mind is that the goal of realist review is increased understanding through middle-range theory. Successful middle-range theories are supported by the data found within the articles included in a realist review, but they are also removed from this data. To illustrate this point further, within a meta-analysis, the results of the meta-analysis are directly related to the data, hence quality control of the "raw" data is very important in order to avoid the problems of "garbage-in equals garbage-out"(Cochrane Collaboration 2006). However as a "layer" of interpretation lies between the data and the middle-range theory in a realist review, there is no direct connection between data quality and middle-range theory. The weak link (if there is one at all) is more at the interpretation level. We thus come to the vexed issue of whose interpretation is more "correct" than the other. In realist reviews, it is not the number of "similar" interpretations that makes the difference (i.e. how many "independent" reviewers undertake each stage) but more the ability of the middle-range theory to explain the data that matters.

A linked matter is that of the transparency and reproducibility of realist reviews. The issue of transparency is an easier one to tackle as we believe that the solution lies in careful documentation of: 1) the review process, with particular attention to documenting and reporting how and why decisions were made; and 2) the "raw" data extracted from our included studies. Ours was a two-year review that included 249 included papers. We felt that we should not be relying on our collective memories when it came to recalling for ourselves and reporting to others how and why key decisions were made. We therefore kept a "research log" of our team meetings and also included in this log notes on how and why key decisions were made during our review. Our use of an Excel spreadsheet and NVivo also greatly assisted us when we had to revisit and resynthesize our data as well as in reporting. Reviewers may wish to make these available to others in a bid to further assist transparency.

The reproducibility issue is much more difficult to address as the results of our review were *our* interpretations of what the data we found meant and how some of it could be accounted for through two middle-range theories. While we are confident that our documentation of our review would provide another review team with all the necessary "raw" data and narrative on our decision-making processes, where interpretation is involved it is always possible that a different review team will come up with a different "take" from the data provided. However, two points are worth raising. In a realist review we fully expect that this might be the case and in fact this is the purpose of our careful documentation. The transparency provided allows for other researchers to use a different "lens" (if they so wish), as we make no claims to the fact that our review is the "gospel truth" and the "last word" on this matter. What we have attempted to do is to "theorize" (Box 5.2) the data in our review to provide a plausible and "successful" series of explanations of the data. One way of viewing the claims from any realist review is that, as with any theory in science, it stands until it is proved wrong or in need of refinement.

Realist reviews are a sense-making process where the success of a review should be based on whether or not sufficient explanation and understanding can be gained through the use of middle-range theory. The fundamental question here is how do you prove a theory is "true"? Our preference is that this is through the "success" of the theory (also sometimes called the Cosmic Coincidence Argument (Klee 1997)). Thus "successful" middle range theory (or theories) from a realist review should be able to explain the demiregularities that are relevant to the research question (with the caveats that a review will necessarily have a specific focus and there may be data limitations).

Theory
Our experience is that many theories often already exist to explain the demiregularities that a review team many encounter in their review. These may be well described and tested or highly speculative. We also found that these

theories may be found in other disciplines. Thus we strongly advise review teams to look beyond their own discipline(s) for both candidate and their "final" middle-range theories. It is, however, always possible there is no pre-existing middle-range theory to explain a middle-range theory and, if this is the case, then a review team should report this and try to develop their own.

Stage 4: drawing conclusions and making recommendations

In this final stage, I have departed from the structure I have used till now. Making recommendations from the findings of a realist review is one of the more challenging aspects of the review process. This relates to the nature of realist reviews. Thus to "set the scene" I have begun with the challenges that a review team faces before moving on to guidance about the process itself.

Challenges

Realist reviewers need to be aware of three challenges when it comes to drawing conclusions and making recommendations. These issues relate to the nature of realist reviews and so I have only focused on the "departures" that realist reviewers need to make (as opposed to making detailed comment on the generalities of how to draw conclusions and make recommendations).

The first relates to the breadth of the claim that can be made. As we have noted in Stage 1, any complex intervention is likely to be amenable to a lifetime's worth of study and so, pragmatically, you have to take a specific focus or "cut" through the literature. Hence any claims that are made should be bound by the "cut" made. For example, we only tested our two middle-range theories on Internet-based education that involved doctors. This does not mean that these are the only two relevant middle-range theories or that these middle-range theories do not operate within other professions. What we can recommend though is that it may be worthwhile searching for other theories and testing our middle-range theories within other professions.

The second issue relates to the data limitations (see Challenges in Stage 3 above). We could not test each and every aspect of our middle-range theories. Thus, at best, we can only ever claim partial understanding of some aspects of the use of the Internet in medical education. We can confidently claim that engagement is an important mechanism and sits squarely at the start of our chain of events (or program theory). We are also confident that after a learner has been engaged, the next step involves the learner using the Internet-based resource(s) to learn. Whilst we know that the CF throws some light on a narrow aspect of this learning (i.e. that it involves dialog with feedback) the rest of the learning mechanism remains a "black box," in that we have not been able to ascertain what else is in this box, and how they are related to one another and finally to the learning outcome (Figure 5.5).

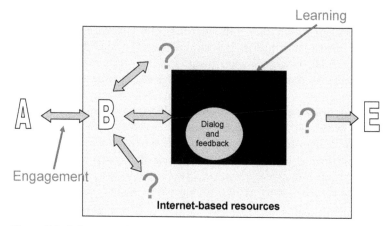

Figure 5.5 A diagrammatic representation of the incomplete causal chain in our review.

The third and final challenge relates to the nature of complex interventions. Human agency is an important "cause" for change in such interventions but human agency is also highly unpredictable. Thus at best, we have demi-regularities and this means that it is not always possible to "predict" what any one (or group of) participants will behave under specific contexts – that is, a context may not always fire the same mechanism in the same way due to the presence and influence of other mechanisms. So once again the strength of any claims made needs to be moderated to reflect the non-deterministic nature of human agency.

Guidance

Based on these three challenges, all realist reviews should best be envisaged as "works in progress" that provide the "best current understanding" about complex interventions. They are never the "last word" or "definitive" and their recommendations or findings should be tested, either on (for example) new or different datasets, or even in empirical trials.

With these three caveats in mind, it is still possible to make recommendations that are potentially useful to researchers, practitioners, patients, and policymakers. In our experience, the main questions that the "consumers" of your review may wish to know are:

- Will it work? We would suggest that this is not the focus of a realist review, which at best is able to answer the question "for whom" it might work. Another systematic review method would seem to be more appropriate (e.g., Cochrane effectiveness review methodology).

- How or why does it work ("active ingredients")?
- When should I use it?
- Whom should I use it for?
- How best can I use it?

The answers to the last four questions will come from your clarification of the chain of events (or program theory) of the complex intervention in question and the middle-range theories that are able to explain the salient demi-regularities that give rise to the outcomes of interest within.

It is worth remembering that the middle-range theories are not only explanatory, but also have some "predictive" powers. Thus, it should be possible to "predict" the ideal (for example) contexts and participants for which a complex intervention might best work bearing in mind the caveat that human agency can never be predicted with absolute certainty. An example of a recommendation to course designers from our review would be; "Learners on all types of Internet-based courses highly value courses that allow them to enter into a dialog with and to get feedback from others (human or virtual) on their performance or understanding. However, course designers will also need to bear in mind that other aspects of courses are also highly valued and act as power factors that will influence learner engagement with a course."

In our review (as you can see from Figure 5.5), we were only able to clearly elucidate the very start of our causal chain and gain an overview of some aspects of the learning process in Internet-based courses in medical education. We chose to present our findings as a series of questions (which were linked directly to components of our "successful" middle-range theories) as we felt that this format might be easier for course developers and learners to use (Box 5.9). In our guidance, our two mechanism engagement and learning are renamed "Engaging learners" and "Achieving interactive dialog" respectively in order to reflect more closely our findings (for example, in that we did not "uncover" every aspect or learning). In the "Engaging learners" section of our guidance we "translated" each attribute (sub-mechanism) from the Innovations Theory into a question. Thus the relative advantage attribute now asks designers and learners to consider the usefulness to them and lists the contexts in which they might find the course useful. This process is repeated for "ease of use" and "compatibility" attributes. Finally, because of our limited findings in our learning mechanism, we restricted our questions in "Achieving interactive dialog" to encouraging designers and participants to think about how dialog and feedback might be operationalized on a course (giving specific examples of techniques drawn from our review).

Box 5.9 Five questions for developers and prospective learners to ask of an Internet-based course

Engaging learners
1 How useful will the prospective learners perceive the Internet technology to be? For example, in any particular context and compared to what is currently available to them, to what extent will this technology:
  a Increase their access to learning?
  b Provide consistent, high-quality content?
  c Be a convenient format in which to receive their education?
  d Save them money?
  e Save them time?
  f Link to course assessment?
2 How easy will the prospective learners find this technology to use?
3 How well does this format fit in with what learners are used to and expect?

Achieving interactive dialog
4 How will high-quality human–human (learner–tutor and learner–learner) interaction be achieved? For example what use will be made of:
  a Structured virtual seminars?
  b Email, bulletin boards?
  c Real-time chat?
  d Supplementary media, e.g. phone calls, videoconferencing?
  e Course assessment and feedback on performance?
5 How will high-quality human–technical interaction be achieved? For example what use will be made of:
  a Questions with automated feedback?
  b Simulations?

Chapter summary

Realist review is best thought of as a type of theory-driven qualitative systematic review method. It has its origins in sociology and is based on the centrality of human agency as the means whereby outcomes come about. In the health sciences, its use has been used mainly to review complex interventions. Within these types of interventions human agency and context have been identified as key factors that determine outcomes thus creating a perfect match of method to intervention type. Realist reviews are thus best suited to the review of the evidence from human agency-mediated interventions. Evidence that may contribute to a realist review can come from almost any source as it has no predetermined hierarchy of evidence.

Realist reviews try not so much to prove that something works, but more to explain "how," "why," "for whom," "in what circumstances," and "to what extent" does it work. The review process is iterative and interpretive and the goal of any realist review is to elucidate the chain of events (or program theory) that leads to outcomes and to explain and understand this through the use of middle-range theory.

Funding and acknowledgements

GW was generously funded to undertake this review by NoCLoR (North Central London Research Consortium, United Kingdom). I am grateful to the following for their help and support whilst undertaking the example realist review: Marcia Rigby (administrative Support), UCL Library (articles retrieval), Trisha Greenhalgh and Ray Pawson (as my supervisors and collaborators), the anonymous peer reviewers of this chapter for their helpful and constructive feedback, and Gill Westhorp for her insights on conceptual clarity.

References

Adams B, Sydie R. (2001) *Sociological Theory*. Thousand Oaks: Pine Forge Press.

Anderson R. (2008) New MRC guidance on evaluating complex interventions. *BMJ*. **337**: a1937.

Cochrane Collaboration. (2009) *Cochrane Handbook for Systematic Reviews of Interventions*. http://www.cochrane.org/resources/handbook/ [accessed 7 June 2011].

Craig P, Dieppe P, Macintyre S, Michie S, Nazareth I, Petticrew M. (2008) Developing and evaluating complex interventions: the new Medical Research Council guidance. *BMJ*. **337**: a1655.

Davis P, McCracken P. (2002) Restructuring rural continuing medical education through videoconferencing. *J Telemed Telecare*. **8**(Suppl 2): 108–9.

Greenhalgh T, Peacock R. (2005) Effectiveness and efficiency of search methods in systematic reviews of complex evidence: audit of primary sources. *BMJ*. **331**: 1064–5.

Greenhalgh T, Kristjansson E, Robinson V. (2007) Realist review to understand the efficacy of school feeding programmes. *BMJ*. **335**(7625): 858–61.

Grundman JA, Wigton RS, Nickol D (2000). A controlled trial of an interactive, web-based virtual reality program for teaching physical diagnosis skills to medical students. *Acad Med*. **75** (10 Suppl): S4–S49.

Haig A, Dozier M. (2003a) BEME Guide No 3: Systematic searching for evidence in medical education - Part 1: Sources of information. *Med Teach*. **25**(4): 352–63.

Haig A, Dozier M. (2003b) BEME Guide No 3: Systematic searching for evidence in medical education - Part 2: Constructing searches. *Med Teach*. **25**(5): 463–84.

Hoban JD, Schlesinger JB, Fairman RP, Grimes MM. (2003) Electrifying a medical school course: a case study. *Teach Learn Med* **15**(2): 140–6.

Huang C. (2003) Changing learning with new interactive and media-rich instruction environments: virtual labs case study report. *Comput Med Imaging Graph*. **27**(2–3): 157–64.

Jao CS, Brint SU, Hier DB. (2005) Making the neurology clerkship more effective: Can e-Textbook facilitate learning? *Neurol Res*. **27**(7): 762–7.

Klee R. (1997) *Introduction to the Philosophy of Science. Cutting Nature at its Seams.* New York: Oxford University Press.

Kroeker KI, Vicas I, Johnson D, Holroyd B, Jennett PA, Johnston RV. (2000) Residency training via videoconference–satisfaction survey. *Telemed J E Health*. **6**(4): 425–8.

Kumar RK, Velan GM, Korell SO, Kandara M, Dee FR, Wakefield D. (2004) Virtual microscopy for learning and assessment in pathology. *J Pathol*. **204**(5): 613–8.

Laurillard D. (2002) *Rethinking University Teaching: A Conversational Framework for the Effective Use of Learning Technologies.* 2nd. ed. London: Routledge Falmer.

Merton R. (1967) *On Theoretical Sociology. Five Essays, Old and New.* New York: The Free Press.

Moore G, Benbasat I. (1991) Development of an instrument to measure the perceptions of adopting an information technology innovation. *Inform Sys Res.* **2**: 192–222.

NVivo 2 (2002) [computer program]. Doncaster, Australia: QSR International.

Pawson R. (2003) Nothing as practical as a good theory. *Evaluation.* **9**(4): 471–90.

Pawson R. (2006) *Evidence-based Policy. A Realist Perspective.* London: Sage.

Pawson R, Tilley N. (1997) *Realistic Evaluation.* London: Sage.

Pawson R, Greenhalgh T, Harvey G, Walshe K. (2005) Realist review – a new method of systematic review designed for complex policy interventions. *J Health Serv Res Policy.* **10**: 21–34.

Reeves T. (2005) Effective dimensions of interactive learning on the world wide web. In: Khan B, editor. *Web-Based Instruction.* 1st ed. Englewood Cliffs, New Jersey: Educational Technology Publications, Inc: pp. 59–66.

Rogers E. (1995) *The Diffusion of Innovations.* 4th ed. New York: Free Press.

Schon D. (1987) *Educating the Reflective Practitioner.* 1st ed. San Francisco, California: Jossey-Bass Inc.

Shepperd S, Lewin L, Straus S, Clarke M, Eccles M, Fitzpatrick R, *et al.* (2009) Can we systematically review studies that evaluate complex interventions? *PLoS Med.* **6**(8): e1000086.

Slotnick H. (1996) How doctors learn: the role of clinical problems across the medical school-to-practice continuum. *Acad Med.* **71**(1): 28–34.

Wong G, Greenhalgh T, Pawson R. (2010) Internet-based medical education: a realist review of what works, for whom and in what circumstances. *BMC Medical Education.* Feb; **10**: 12.

Chapter 6 **Mixed methods synthesis: a worked example**

Josephine Kavanagh, BA, MA[1], Fiona Campbell[2], Angela Harden, PhD[3], and James Thomas, PhD[1]

[1]*EPPI-Centre, Social Science Research Unit, Institute of Education, University of London, London, UK*
[2]*School of Health and Related Research, University of Sheffield, Sheffield, UK*
[3]*Institute for Health and Human Development, School of Health and Biosciences, University of East London, London, UK*

The issue of integrating both qualitative and quantitative data has grown in importance. Systematic reviews of complex social and public health interventions increasingly address questions that go beyond "what works" and ask "what works – for whom – and under what circumstances?" Answering these broader questions requires the inclusion of qualitative studies in research synthesis which address the understanding, attitudes, behaviors, and experiences of the targets of interventions. While there is a strong body of research on methods for reviewing quantitative and qualitative evidence, methods to enable the synthesis of the two remain less well developed. A mixed methods approach to research synthesis developed by researchers at the EPPI-Centre is described here. Three distinct stages of the review process support the integration of two epistemologically diverse traditions. The first stage is a traditional systematic review of effectiveness (with or without meta-analysis); the second a synthesis of qualitative research which addresses questions of intervention need, implementation, acceptability, and appropriateness; and, finally a cross-study synthesis which brings the findings of both earlier syntheses together. For stage two a thematic synthesis is proposed by the authors. Thematic synthesis builds upon the techniques of grounded-theory and meta-ethnography. It involves: the coding of text "line-by-line;" the development of descriptive themes; and the generation of "analytical themes." Implications for interventions are derived from the analytical themes and are linked to the findings of the effectiveness review in the final cross-study synthesis. This final stage is a comparative analysis which juxtaposes the findings of both syntheses to identify appropriate and acceptable interventions which match the needs and experiences of those targeted by interventions. The mixed

Synthesizing Qualitative Research: Choosing the Right Approach, First Edition.
Edited by Karin Hannes and Craig Lockwood.
© 2012 John Wiley & Sons, Ltd. Published 2012 by John Wiley & Sons, Ltd.

methods approach is illustrated in a case example of a systematic review of dietary and physical activity interventions for weight management in pregnancy. This review found that important factors that influence maternal weight gain were not addressed by the intervention studies, such as: the difficulty women encounter when seeking to use gym facilities when pregnant and the conflict between lay health beliefs held by the wider family and healthy eating messages.

Introduction

Earlier chapters have described a range of methods for qualitative evidence synthesis, summarizing how qualitative synthesis can contribute to evidence-informed policy and practice decision-making across a number of fields. In this chapter we describe an approach to integrating both quantitative and qualitative research in systematic reviews using a mixed methods approach. This approach combines the statistical meta-analysis of the findings from trials to answer questions about "what works?" with the thematic synthesis of the findings from qualitative research to address questions of experience, process, and context. The methods described in this chapter were developed by researchers at the Evidence for Policy and Practice Information and Co-ordinating (EPPI) Centre, in the Social Science Research Unit at the Institute of Education, University of London in the UK (Harden & Thomas 2005; Oliver et al. 2005; Thomas et al. 2004), and have since been endorsed and adopted by other researchers and research groups around the world (e.g. Chalmers 2005; Ely et al. 2007; Roberts & Noyes 2009). The resulting systematic reviews are a type of mixed methods systematic review that has been defined as combining "the findings of qualitative and quantitative studies within a single review in order to address overlapping or complementary questions" (Harden & Thomas 2010, p. 750). In this chapter we describe in more detail the origins and theoretical underpinnings of the method, outline the steps involved, and provide a worked example to illustrate the method in action. The review used as the worked example was led by a team at the University of Sheffield in the UK and was conducted independently of the team who developed the mixed methods approach. We end the chapter with some reflections on the strengths and challenges of this approach to integrating qualitative and quantitative research in systematic reviews.

Origins and theoretical assumptions

The mixed methods approach to integrating qualitative and quantitative research in systematic reviews described in this chapter was developed within an EPPI-Centre programme of work on evidence-based health promotion and public health funded by the English Department of Health. Initially, policymakers sought systematic reviews addressing intervention effectiveness.

However, questions about "what works?" were soon supplemented with questions about "what works – for whom – and under what circumstances," as well as questions about health needs, appropriateness, and acceptability. Answering these questions required the inclusion of what is often described as "qualitative" research, and, in particular, research that reported the perspectives and experiences of the population groups that health promotion and public health interventions are targeted at. We began to use the term "views" studies as a shorthand to describe these largely qualitative studies, because they shared a central characteristic – the primary focus being one that privileges the views and experiences of participants themselves to uncover their worldview. Including qualitative research in systematic reviews of effectiveness posed a significant challenge to the EPPI-Centre team, who embarked on this work in 1999, in that no standard method or template for the quality assessment and synthesis of qualitative research alongside trials in systematic reviews had yet emerged.

The teams' starting point for the synthesis of qualitative research and its integration with quantitative research was to adapt the standard systematic review model designed to answer questions of effectiveness – developed and promoted with great success by, for example, the Cochrane Collaboration – and to draw on methods already established for data analysis in primary qualitative research. In their adaptation of the standard systematic review model the team worked with several key principles: transparency (to be explicit about the methods used to integrate different types of studies); error avoidance (to use strategies to enhance the rigor of our reviews); user involvement (to consult and negotiate with policymakers at several points throughout the review process to ensure that the review would be relevant as well as scientifically robust); matching and adapting review methods according to the study type under review; a complementary rather than competing view of qualitative and quantitative research; and a commitment to learning from the experiences of the intended targets of the policies and practices under review.

The systematic review and synthesis of qualitative research *and* its integration with quantitative research are not without controversy and epistemological conundrums. Some qualitative researchers oppose the synthesis of qualitative findings outright, arguing that combining findings from different studies would divorce findings from their original research context. Other qualitative researchers support the synthesis of findings across multiple studies but argue that the traditional systematic review framework is a "quantitative" enterprise that is not appropriate for the review of "qualitative" research (e.g., Dixon-Woods *et al.* 2006a). There are echoes of the paradigm wars in this position whereby the qualitative and quantitative research paradigms are seen as incommensurable because of fundamental epistemological differences. From this view there is little point in integrating qualitative and quantitative research. As Guba (1987, p. 31) notes, one paradigm precludes the other "just as surely as the belief in a round world precludes belief in a flat one." However, as Creswell (2010, p. 54) argues, the "paradigm debate," which asserted that work undertaken in different paradigms cannot be mixed, has diminished in recent years and there are now a range of "paradigm stances" that researchers can adopt when mixing methods, such as a the complementary strengths stance (whereby the paradigms are seen as different rather than incompatible, but because they are different they should be kept separate in mixed methods research) or an alternative paradigm stance (whereby a single paradigm provides the foundation for integrating the research, and this foundation may be found in, for example, pragmatism or a transformative-emancipatory perspective). Our starting paradigm stance for mixed methods systematic reviews was a complementary strengths one.

In a recent critical overview of methods for qualitative research synthesis, Barnet-Page and Thomas (2009) constructed a useful typology of synthesis methods based on their epistemological foundations. The typology divides synthesis methods into two broad camps: idealist, that err more toward social constructivist viewpoints; and realist, that assume the existence of an external reality, albeit with the acceptance that research can only ever be a representation of that reality. Idealist approaches are characterized by being flexible in their approach to identifying and assessing the quality of the literature they contain, and are more likely to aim to locate it within its disciplinary context. Examples of idealist approaches are critical interpretive synthesis (Dixon-Woods *et al.* 2006b) and meta-narrative mapping (Greenhalgh *et al.* 2005). Realist approaches follow methods that are similar to the traditional systematic review with prespecified search strategies and predetermined inclusion and quality criteria. In addition, they are less likely to use the paradigm within which the primary research was conducted as part of their analysis. The epistemological foundation of our approach to the synthesis of qualitative research is towards the realist end of the idealist–realist continuum.

Steps in a mixed methods approach

The mixed methods approach has three distinct elements or stages that enable learning to be integrated from two epistemologically diverse traditions. The first element is a traditional systematic review of intervention effectiveness (with or without meta-analysis); the second a synthesis to address related questions of process, context of meaning using qualitative research, and

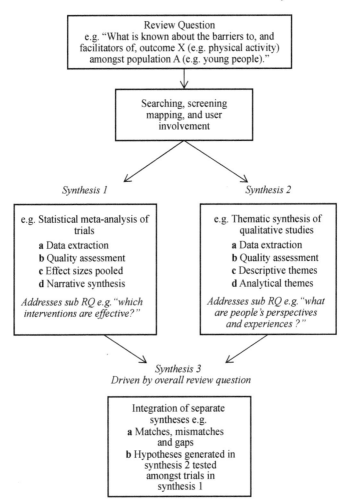

Figure 6.1 A mixed methods approach to conducting a systematic review of diverse study types. Reproduced from Harden A, Garcia J, Oliver S, Rees R, Shepherd J, Brunton G, Oakley A, Applying systematic review methods to studies of people's views: an example from public health, *Journal of Epidemiology and Community Health* **58**: 794–800, 2004, with permission from BMJ Publishing Group Ltd.

finally a cross study synthesis (Figure 6.1). As noted above, a key principle underpinning this mixed methods approach are that it should maintain the existing principles of systematic reviews, remaining question driven, transparent, and where possible and appropriate, select, appraise, and synthesize all research evidence relevant to the question(s).

The effectiveness synthesis

The first synthesis aims to address questions about the effects of interventions and to estimate the balance of benefit and harm from the intervention(s) under review. The effectiveness synthesis follows established methods for systematic reviews of intervention effects incorporating statistical meta-analysis when appropriate. These methods have been described in great detail elsewhere and are not repeated here (e.g., Egger *et al.* 2001; Higgins & Green 2009; Lipsey & Wilson 2001). Following exhaustive searching, systematic screening, quality appraisal, and data extraction the effect sizes from trials are pooled. Variation (heterogeneity) may be explored using subgroup analyses on a limited range of categories, specified in advance (e.g., study quality, study design, setting, and type of intervention). Exploratory narrative analysis may also be used to compare characteristics of interventions showing harmful effects, no effects, or positive effects. Such an analysis can reveal several potential explanations for heterogeneity in effects, but these must be viewed as speculative since it is difficult to avoid data dredging with this type of analysis.

The qualitative synthesis

The second synthesis aims to address different questions, albeit questions related to effectiveness, such as those about intervention context, implementation, appropriateness, acceptability, and need. In EPPI-Centre reviews these questions have frequently been framed around the perspectives and experiences of the intended recipients of interventions under review. Thematic synthesis – a synthesis method developed within EPPI-Centre reviews (Thomas & Harden 2008) – has often been used in the centre's reviews to synthesize the qualitative (and other types of) research that examine perspectives and experiences. Other researchers adopting our mixed methods approach have used other qualitative synthesis methods such as meta-ethnography.

Thematic synthesis (Box 6.1) builds upon some of the principles and techniques from meta-ethnography (Noblit & Hare 1988) and grounded theory (Strauss & Corbin, 1998), and has been facilitated through the use of the web-based systematic review software EPPI-Reviewer (Thomas *et al.* 2010). The term "thematic synthesis" has been employed to acknowledge that this synthesis method builds upon methods for thematic analysis for primary qualitative research. The "raw data" for this synthesis are the text from study reports that are labeled by the authors as "findings" or "results." These data are to some extent interpretative, however as described earlier, a primary focus of "views" studies is to privilege the views and experiences of the research participants.

Box 6.1 Steps in a thematic synthesis (based on Thomas & Harden 2008)

Stages one and two: coding text and developing descriptive themes
The first stage of a thematic synthesis involves the identification of themes across the included studies. This aims to be a fairly descriptive activity, remaining "close" to the data and encapsulating the studies' findings in a framework that relates the themes they contain to one another. The following, analytical stage, aims to draw conclusions from the findings of stage one, in the light of the conceptual framework of the review and its review questions.

Identifying the "findings"
The first task in stage one is to identify the "findings" of the primary studies. Findings can appear almost anywhere in a paper or report (and it is possible to conceptualize the whole report as "findings"). As we are usually concerned with identifying what people think, feel, or believe about a given phenomenon, we often look for sections in papers that report what participants say (both individually and corporately). Thematic syntheses can also use the conclusions of primary reports, depending on their given objectives. We acknowledge, however, that all thematic synthesis is essentially an interpretation of primary reports, which are themselves authors' interpretations of what study participants were saying. Once the "findings" have been identified, they are entered verbatim into standard software for undertaking qualitative analysis (e.g. NVivo or Atlas TI) or specialist reviewing software (e.g., EPPI-Reviewer).

Line-by-line coding
Using a method familiar to those involved in analyzing primary research, each line of text from the primary studies is then assigned one or more codes than encapsulate its meaning. As soon as codes begin to be applied to a second study, the task of *conceptual translation* has begun: a key characteristic of the synthesis of qualitative research. This involves identifying concepts that studies have in common, though they may be expressed in different words. Noblit and Hare outline two aspects of this: *reciprocal* and *refutational* translation, in which concepts are identified as supporting or dissenting from one another. The use of line-by-line coding ensures that a link between the descriptive codes and the primary studies on which they are derived is maintained, and also that they are used consistently across studies.

Developing descriptive themes
Either as part of the process of generating descriptive codes or once it is complete, reviewers then organize their emerging findings into *descriptive themes*. This involves developing an overarching conceptual framework that groups conceptually similar codes and may appear similar to the development of a theory about how study participants perceive the phenomena under discussion. Though this framework is the interpretation of the reviewers who generated it, it should nevertheless aim to summarize what the primary studies said, rather than drawing new and original conclusions. In some reviews, the synthetic activity will stop at this point, since the descriptive themes answer the review questions satisfactorily; some reviews require an additional, more analytical, stage.

Stage three: generating analytical themes
The final activity in a thematic synthesis is the (optional) generation of analytical themes. These themes explicitly take the synthesis "beyond" the content of the primary study, and generate new interpretive conclusions. They are generated in an iterative process. First, each area – and possibly each theme – in the descriptive synthesis are considered *in the light of the review's research questions.* Reviewers ask the question "how does this theme address/answer this question?" and record the result as a statement. (In the first review in which we generated this method, these statements were the barriers to, and facilitators of, healthy eating among children.) A second thematic analysis is then applied to these statements to draw out the cross-cutting *analytical themes* that they contain. These themes and statements are the final product of a thematic synthesis and can later be used to interrogate trials in the mixed methods synthesis.

The data for the synthesis are entered verbatim into a qualitative analysis software package and subjected to thematic synthesis. Thematic synthesis is conducted in three main stages: (1) the coding of text "line-by-line," (2) the development of "descriptive themes," and (3) the generation of "analytical themes." The starting point for the first two stages of the analysis is the findings of the studies themselves without necessarily any direct reference to the questions of the review. The review questions do, however, drive the third stage, when analytical themes are generated, and this is a crucial step in the preparation for the third cross-study synthesis. From the analytical themes, a set of implications for interventions can be derived that helps to link the findings of the qualitative synthesis to the effectiveness synthesis. In the worked example provided, implications for policy and intervention development were reached through a consensus method involving the reviewers and stake-holders (patient groups, commissioners of review, and experts).

Cross-study synthesis
The analytical themes and associated implications for interventions are the starting point for the integration of the "qualitative" and "quantitative" phases of the review. The integration is carried out in two main stages. First, all of the interventions evaluated by the trials are assessed for the extent to which they address or incorporate the implications for interventions derived from the qualitative synthesis. The results of this analysis can be charted within a conceptual and methodological matrix that plots the implications for interventions against the trials. This enables the identification of interventions that match or address the implications for interventions derived from the qualitative synthesis, those that represent a mismatch, and research gaps.

This kind of comparative analysis, which juxtaposes the findings from the first synthesis against the findings of the second, identifies appropriate and acceptable interventions that capture the needs and experiences of those targeted by interventions. The analysis also reveals aspects of those needs and experiences that have been ignored (or were unknown) by those developing and evaluating interventions.

The cross-study synthesis can be pushed one step further in situations where there are sufficient numbers of well-evaluated interventions that either match or do not match the implications for interventions derived from the qualitative synthesis. In these situations, the effect sizes of those interventions that address and those that do not address the implications for interventions can be compared. Standard statistical tests can be conducted to test whether interventions that did address the implications for interventions had a bigger effect than those that did not. Caution is, however, advised in interpreting the findings of these tests; the method might be considered to be a good way of generating hypotheses for future interventions to test, rather than for determining critical policy or practice decisions.

A worked example

We have chosen to illustrate the stages and methods of a mixed methods systematic review using a systematic review of dietary and physical activity interventions for weight management in pregnancy. This review was conducted by researchers from Sheffield University in the UK, and was commissioned to provide evidence to support public health guidance produced by the National Institute of Health and Clinical Excellence (NICE) in England. This review aimed to systematically review evidence of the effectiveness, acceptability, and feasibility of dietary and physical activity interventions for weight management in pregnancy. It is an excellent example of how a mixed methods approach can provide policymakers with evidence of how the contextual factors which surround intervention delivery can influence intervention effectiveness. For example researchers sought to examine how the intervention setting, intervention provider, or personal and social beliefs and views of pregnant women (and their families and healthcare providers) about diet, physical activity, and weight management in pregnancy might influence intervention effectiveness.

In this section we describe the background to the review and how the team conducted the review, focusing in particular on the decision-making that went on throughout the process of developing the questions for the review; drawing up the review protocol and other preparatory work; searching for relevant studies; appraising quality; extracting data; and synthesis.

Background to the review and question development

Excessive weight gain in pregnancy is an important public health concern in the UK and elsewhere. For example, in the UK approximately 20 per cent of pregnant women are obese, and 43 per cent gain excessive weight (Kanagalingam *et al.* 2005). Women who are overweight or obese have an increased risk of a range of complications during pregnancy and childbirth, including: miscarriage, pre-eclampsia, thromboembolism, gestational diabetes, post-partum haemorrhage, induction of labour, instrumental birth, and caesarean section. Furthermore, it has been reported that being overweight and obesity in pregnancy can be directly or indirectly associated with over half of all maternal deaths in the UK (Lewis 2007). There are also increased risks to the fetus of macrosomia, congential anomaly, and intrauterine death (Lewis 2007). Given the identifiable health risks to both mother and child of being overweight or obese during pregnancy, a clear evidence-based policy about the best ways to manage weight gain prior to and in pregnancy for all women whether of normal weight, overweight, or obese was required. Synthesizing trials testing the effectiveness of interventions to prevent excessive weight gain would form a key part of the evidence-base.

It was important, however, to also consider the complexities in the epidemiological evidence and the social context of obesity, weight gain, and eating. The observed relationship between pregnancy, obesity, and health risks is not completely clear: some research suggests that other determinants, such as socioeconomic status and ethnicity, may be confounding the reported association of excessive weight in pregnancy and poor perinatal outcomes (Sheiner *et al.* 2004). Obesity is a socially constructed issue and eating is a social activity (Crossley 2004). Further, social inequalities may contribute to differing perceptions of obesity, food, and nutrition. A recent study of middle- and low-income women's experiences of motherhood and food noted that weight loss is valued differently by different classes of women; that being a mother means putting the needs of the family above the self; and that one-size-fits-all health promotion-based weight loss approaches discretely focused on food, bodies, and eating are "disembodied and disengaged from the social contexts in which people live their lives" (Warin *et al.* 2008, p. 98). These findings illustrate important differences in the way in which diverse groups of women may approach weight gain over their childbearing years. These differences may influence the success of dietary or physical activity interventions for pregnant women.

Understanding more about diverse groups of women's experiences of maintaining their weight during pregnancy through the inclusion of qualitative research in the review was hypothesized by the review team and review commissioners to be able to add depth to understanding why interventions are effective and how to ensure that they are delivered in an acceptable and appropriate manner. This understanding was also anticipated to contribute to the development of interventions yet to be evaluated which address women's understanding of what helps and hinders healthy weight management in pregnancy.

The questions of the review were therefore posed as:

1 What is the effectiveness of interventions to prevent excessive weight gain in pregnancy?
2 What are the perspectives and experiences of pregnant women around weight, diet and physical activity?
3 What factors may influence intervention effectiveness?

A quantitative approach was applied to question 1 while question 2 was asked from a qualitative perspective drawing on the views of women. Question 3 combines both qualitative and quantitative perspectives.

Preparatory work and protocol development

The review team decided to adopt the mixed methods approach to reviewing developed by the EPPI-centre for a number of reasons. The team viewed the approach as well explained and transparent making it ideal for them to pick up and use easily. There was flexibility in the method as it allowed for the inclusion of a range of "quantitative" and "qualitative" studies. The opportunity the method presents to create a dialog between the qualitative and quantitative studies also made this approach appealing especially in relation to addressing the third question of the review.

A protocol was developed by the reviewers in close dialog with a wider consultation team including review commissioners, content experts, policymakers, and consumers. This ensured that the review scope was defined collaboratively and addressed the issues that were important to various stakeholders. The protocol facilitated consultation with relevant stakeholders on the search strategy so that all the relevant search terms, databases, and key journals that would assist in a comprehensive search for relevant research could be defined. The consultation team was also asked to identify relevant papers they were aware of.

The protocol was written according to standard systematic review headings with subheadings to describe separate methods and processes for the effectiveness part of the review and the qualitative part. For example, we set up distinct sets of inclusion criteria for trials and for qualitative studies (Box 6.2).

Box 6.2 Inclusion criteria for studies in a mixed methods review of weight management interventions in pregnancy

Quantitative studies	Qualitative studies
Inclusion criteria	Inclusion criteria
• RCTs (including cluster randomized trials)	• Qualitative studies providing evidence regarding the views of pregnant women, their partners and families, service providers, including practitioners delivering antenatal services, regarding diet, physical activity, and weight management in pregnancy
• Published in English	
• Women aged 18 or over, pregnant or planning a pregnancy; normal weight, overweight, or obese	
• Interventions which included dietary and/or physical activity interventions	• Qualitative studies were taken to be studies which used techniques such as in-depth interviews, focus groups, observation, reflective diaries and case-study methodologies to explore participants experiences
	• Qualitative evidence collected within RCTS included in the effectiveness part of the review as well as relevant stand-alone qualitative studies
Exclusion criteria	Exclusion criteria
• Women with underlying medical conditions	• Studies conducted outside of the UK
• Women expecting more than one baby	
• Underweight women (BMI <18.5 kg/m^2)	
• Studies conducted in a non-OECD countries	

Search

A comprehensive search of both published and unpublished "gray literature" was undertaken to identify relevant studies and background information. Eleven databases were searched and the citation list of relevant review articles and included papers were also searched. The searches were undertaken in early December 2008 and a second search, updating the first, was conducted in August 2009.

The search strategy was not restricted by study design, which facilitated the identification of the diverse range of study designs required for the review. More commonly systematic reviews include a search filter to identify specific study designs, such as a randomized controlled trials (in reviews of clinical effects) or qualitative studies (in qualitative systematic reviews). Searches were limited by year of publication (1990–2008), corresponding with the introduction of the concept of excessive gestational weight gain by the IOM (1990) when it published recommended guidance for gestational weight gain. Where possible limits were applied to retrieve studies in humans and English language citations only.

The search strategy combined terms for pregnancy and terms for body composition, obesity, and weight change. This set of "population" terms was then combined with terms for diet, exercise, physical activity advice, and monitoring, giving four separate sets of results for each database. In addition a bibliographic search of all the included studies was carried out and experts in the field were also consulted to identify any additional literature.

The search results were screened independently by one reviewer and all excluded references were checked by a second reviewer. Where insufficient information was present in the title and abstract to determine eligibility, full papers were retrieved for further consideration. This process was more time-consuming because of the search for qualitative studies. Frequently there was insufficient information from the title to indicate whether an article reported a qualitative research study or whether it was simply an opinion piece. Consequently relatively few qualitative papers could be excluded at the initial title sifting stage. All potentially eligible studies were obtained and re-assessed for inclusion. The inclusion of any studies that were unclear was resolved through discussion.

The search and screening process resulted in the identification of five trials and eight qualitative studies.

Quality appraisal

The selection of appropriate tools to judge quality of included studies and how to incorporate the quality assessment in the analysis of data remains an area of ongoing debate and research. Different tools were used to assess the quality of trials and the qualitative studies. The internal validity of each included trial was assessed using the Cochrane Collaboration's tool for assessing risk of bias. This tool was used because it assesses aspects of trial design that have been empirically shown to influence the validity and reliability of the trial outcomes. The tool assesses six key methodological domains: sequence generation, allocation concealment, baseline comparability, intention to treat analysis, and loss to follow-up and selective outcome reporting.

The use of assessment tools to critically appraise qualitative studies is also an area of evolving methodology (Noyes *et al.* 2008). Qualitative studies encompass a wide breadth of research methodologies limiting the applicability of generic appraisal criteria (Dixon-Woods *et al.* 2004). In this example the reviewers adopted the quality assessment tool for qualitative studies included in the NICE Methods Manual (National Institute for Health and Clinical Excellence 2006). This tool drew on a range of qualitative checklists and designed questions exploring the theoretical approach adopted, methods of sampling, rigor in data collection, exploration of the role of the researcher in the review, description of the context, reliability of methods and analysis, rigor of data analysis, richness of data, coherence of findings, and consideration of relevant ethical issues.

Data extraction

Separate data extraction forms were developed for the trials and qualitative studies in consultation with clinical experts and each was piloted. For the trials, data on study methods, characteristics of participants, interventions, and relevant outcomes were independently extracted by two reviewers from included trials. Any differences in data extraction were resolved by discussion. Data extraction of the qualitative studies was undertaken somewhat differently. Each study, after being read initially to confirm that it fulfilled the inclusion criteria, was then subjected to repeated independent readings during which it was appraised and its findings summarized on the data extraction form (Box 6.3). Consideration was given to the ways in which the methodologies used shaped understandings about the subject of interest (in this case barriers and facilitators affecting healthy weight management in pregnancy).

Box 6.3 Qualitative data extraction form

Review Details
Author, year
Reference ID
Publication type (ie full report or abstract)
Country of corresponding author
Language of publication
Sources of funding
Study design
Authors' objective(s) of review
Methodological Characteristics
Population
Setting
Inclusion/exclusion criteria
Method of recruitment
Method of data collection
Method of data analysis
Theoretical assumptions/definitions of concepts

Clinical Issues
Measures
Comparators
Definition of outcomes
Results
Total number of participants
Participants' baseline characteristics (age, gender, ethnicity, co-morbidities, previous drinking levels)
Duration of study
Findings 1
Findings 2
Authors' comments on strengths/weaknesses of review
Summary
Authors' overall conclusions
Quality assessment of review
Generalizability to UK
Reviewer's comments

Data synthesis

The data synthesis was conducted in three stages according to the mixed methods framework described above.

Effectiveness synthesis

First, where possible and if appropriate, the results of the RCTs were statistically synthesized in a meta-analysis to assess the effectiveness of the interventions in the controlled trials. Meta-analysis was undertaken using Cochrane Collaboration Review Manager 5.0 software. The mean difference was used to estimate the pooled mean difference in weight gained between intervention and control groups, using a random effects model. Statistical heterogeneity between trials was assessed using the chi^2 test, its corresponding P-value and the I^2 test. Sensitivity analyses were performed excluding poor quality trials. Subgroup analyses were performed grouping trials into pre-specified categories. Subgroup analyses according to baseline BMI status or type of intervention (e.g., impact of using regular weight monitoring with feedback to participants) did not demonstrate any difference in the effect of the intervention. The small number of studies limited the exploration of the effects of different features of the interventions.

The main finding of this synthesis was that there was no significant evidence that dietary interventions with or without additional support to increase physical activity were effective in reducing gestational weight gain (Figure 6.2).

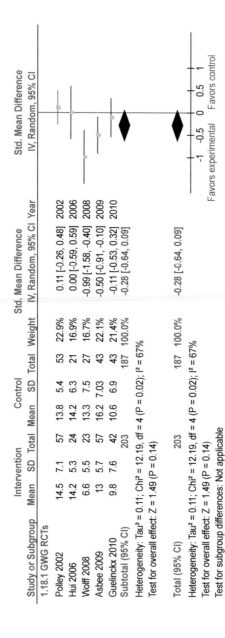

The following content corresponds to the forest plot figure:

| Study or Subgroup | Intervention | | | Control | | | Weight | Std. Mean Difference IV, Random, 95% CI | Year |
	Mean	SD	Total	Mean	SD	Total			
1.18.1 GWG RCTs									
Polley 2002	14.5	7.1	57	13.8	5.4	53	22.9%	0.11 [-0.26, 0.48]	2002
Hui 2006	14.2	5.3	24	14.2	6.3	21	16.9%	0.00 [-0.59, 0.59]	2006
Wolff 2008	6.6	5.5	23	13.3	7.5	27	16.7%	-0.99 [-1.58, -0.40]	2008
Asbee 2009	13	5.7	57	16.2	7.03	43	22.1%	-0.50 [-0.91, -0.10]	2009
Guelinckx 2010	9.8	7.6	42	10.6	6.9	43	21.4%	-0.11 [-0.53, 0.32]	2010
Subtotal (95% CI)			203			187	100.0%	-0.28 [-0.64, 0.09]	

Heterogeneity: Tau² = 0.11; Chi² = 12.19, df = 4 (P = 0.02); I² = 67%
Test for overall effect: Z = 1.49 (P = 0.14)

Total (95% CI)			203			187	100.0%	-0.28 [-0.64, 0.09]	

Heterogeneity: Tau² = 0.11; Chi² = 12.19, df = 4 (P = 0.02); I² = 67%
Test for overall effect: Z = 1.49 (P = 0.14)
Test for subgroup differences: Not applicable

Favors experimental   Favors control

Figure 6.2 Results of the statistical meta-analysis of trials in a mixed methods review of weight management interventions in pregnancy. Reproduced from Campbell F, Johnson M, Messina J, *et al.* Behavioural interventions for weight management in pregnancy: A systematic review of quantitative and qualitative data. *BMC Public Health* 2011, **11**:491 doi:10.1186/1471-2458-11-491

Synthesis of qualitative research

Second, thematic analysis of the findings from the qualitative studies was conducted. As noted earlier, each of the five studies were read and re-read to enable the reviewer to familiarize themselves with the studies. Findings were summarized on the data extraction form and consideration was given to the ways in which the methodologies used shaped understandings about the subject of interest (in this case barriers and facilitators affecting healthy weight management in pregnancy). After repeated readings and summarizing of the findings, common themes were identified and supporting quotes drawn from the qualitative studies. One reviewer undertook this process.

Women expressed many different views and attitudes to diet, physical activity, and weight gain in pregnancy. Three themes emerged in the analysis of these studies relating to women's views of weight management in pregnancy: contradictory messages, pregnancy as a time of transition, and change and a perceived lack of control (Figure 6.3).

Cross-study synthesis

The final step was to bring the findings of the synthesis of the qualitative and quantitative systematic reviews together in order to discover to what extent interventions addressed the factors that influence gestational weight gain (Box 6.4).

We constructed a methodological and conceptual matrix to integrate the findings of the two syntheses. The potential implications of the views of pregnant women, their partners, families, and health professionals for interventions were presented alongside the content and findings of the interventions evaluated by the trials. Matches and gaps were identified. Potential mismatches were explored but not found.

An example of a match was the implication from the qualitative research that interventions address the contradictory nature of advice and information on healthy eating and physical activity during pregnancy. This was addressed by all the interventions evaluated by the trials. Despite this, however, the interventions were not shown to be effective. Drawing on the findings of the qualitative synthesis, one explanation might be the powerful influence on women's behavior of their peer support system which may undermine the messages of health professionals. Interventions at a community level may support interventions that are targeting the behavior of individual pregnant women.

An example of a gap was that the interventions included in the trials did not seek to address the wider, social factors that might contribute to poor weight management. Pregnancy was a time of change and transition for women.

Theme	Description
Contradictory messages	• Advice and information from health professionals, peers, and family often seen as contradictory and confusing ("There's no black and white about what you should and shouldn't do so I don't, I can't follow it at all" (Gross & Bee 2004, p. 165)) • Women reported strong encouragement from peers to rest and to increase their intake of certain food types, such as milk and cheese • Professionals were often reluctant to initiate discussion around weight management due to fear of "victimizing" women
Pregnancy as a time of transition and change	• Needs of unborn child take precedence over mothers • Decline in physical activity and increase in eating – these behavior patterns reinforced by social networks and environment • Changing body image: positive ("now I have a wonderful excuse to be big" (Fox & Yamguchi 1997, p. 38)) and negative ("fat," "bloated," and "frumpy")
Perceived lack of control	• Weight gain as inevitable ("It's just one of those things that you expect happens when you are pregnant, you almost hand your body over to these people and you just accept whatever they say or do to you without really questioning it." (Warriner, 2000, p. 621)) • Restricted access to gym and normal physical activities • Physical demands of pregnancy restricted activity and influenced dietary patterns

Figure 6.3 Overview of themes from the synthesis of qualitative research in a mixed methods review of weight management in pregnancy.

Some described it as a time when they felt a loss of control over their bodies, a time of transition, after which normal patterns of dietary limitation and exercise would resume. Facilitating behavior change may be more effective amongst women where a sense of control is felt and interventions delivered in such a way as to re-establish this sense of control. All of the interventions evaluated by the trials assumed compliance with the underlying values implicit within them – that is that weight gain and being overweight is not good. For some women these may be attitudes that are hard to accept, pregnancy may be a time when they feel comfortable, able to eat with fewer limitations, and find being overweight being more socially acceptable. As such, health messages may not have been accepted and adopted by participants.

The pattern of convergence and divergence between the interventions and the factors identified in the qualitative studies may explain the mixed results

Box 6.4 Synthesis matrix

Potential barriers and facilitators to healthy weight management in pregnancy	Extent to which these were addressed in the trials
Diet and exercise – factors external to the individual.	
Access to adequate and relevant information and advice was somewhat ad-hoc. Information from health professionals was often vague or contradictory.	All of the intervention studies except Kardel and Kase (1997) addressed this factor by delivering interventions that provided clear and consistent advice to pregnant women often using different methods to reinforce health messages.
Women accessed information and advice relating to weight management from three main sources; healthcare professionals, family and friends, and the media.	None of the studies sought to influence the other sources of information that influence women's behavior in pregnancy. Nor did they describe methods of supporting women who may be hearing conflicting messages from differing sources.
There were practical barriers to exercise with women finding that gyms did not encourage participation by pregnant women.	The focus of the interventions was at the level of the individual and did not seek to influence beliefs regarding pregnancy and the need to maintain exercise as a part of effective weight management in pregnancy in the wider community.
A lack of exercise provision actually targeting pregnant women with midwifery support.	Four studies offered exercise classes as part of the intervention (Hui *et al.* 2006; Kinnunen *et al.* 2007; Claaesson 2007; and Gray Donald 2000).
Diet and exercise factors specific to the individual.	
Appetites and food preferences were disrupted in pregnancy.	Apart from Guelinckx *et al.*, (2008) all of the interventions offered tailored advice which may have incorporated women's preferences.
For some who were already overweight before pregnancy, pregnancy was a time when they felt it was legitimate to be overweight and their self-esteem was higher as a result.	Individually targeted interventions will not challenge the cultural values surrounding body shape, though they may assist women in making informed choices and in resisting unhelpful discourses.

Women's attitudes and behaviors in relation to diet and physical activity during pregnancy are associated with pre-pregnancy attitudes and behavior to diet and exercise.	Only one case report described an intervention for overweight women trying to get pregnant (Galletly et al. 1996). All of the other interventions specifically targeted interventions during pregnancy.
For some women pregnancy is a time when women feel it is legitimate to relax on self-imposed dietary limitations and weight gain can be dealt with later.	This was not reported in the interventions described.
For some women weight gain in pregnancy is regarded as a norm and excessive weight gain can be addressed once they are no longer pregnant.	Use of regular monitoring of weight and plotting of weight on graphs combined with stepped care would challenge this view.
Women's experiences of and attitudes to body image fluctuate during pregnancy.	It may be difficult to map the timing of interventions effectively onto the fluctuating subjectivities of pregnant women.
Conflicting lay beliefs. A perception that eating was a way of protecting the baby and a woman should be "eating for two."	The interventions will have addressed the mothers lay beliefs but not the beliefs of important significant others who will give conflicting messages.
There were many barriers to exercise in pregnancy including physical discomfort experienced by women, important lay messages about the need for rest, and pregnancy offering a legitimate reason for not being active. Perceived risks associated with exercise might be appropriate (facilitator) or inappropriate (barrier) compared to guidance.	The barriers to exercise were only partially addressed by the interventions. They conveyed messages about the safety of exercise in pregnancy and some offered classes for women to attend.

seen in the outcomes of the intervention studies. No clear pattern of effectiveness emerged and this would suggest that other important factors are influencing maternal weight gain in pregnancies which are not being sufficiently addressed in the interventions reviewed here.

Strengths and challenges of the approach

The EPPI-Centre method of integrating qualitative and quantitative findings offered a transparent and coherent approach that we could adopt readily despite little experience of integrating qualitative and quantitative studies in previous systematic reviews. The final stage of the analysis, incorporating results into a matrix with the results from each arm of the review, juxtaposed facilitated in-depth analysis about the implications of the findings and how they illuminated the hidden complexities of why interventions might and might not work within different contexts. This analysis was also positive in informing recommendations about the direction for future research.

The added value that the mixed methods approach brought to the review did come at a cost. A mixed methods approach to review is resource intensive. Traditional systematic reviews usually involve one type of study and one type of synthesis whereas the mixed methods approach reported here involves three ("sub-") syntheses and two main study types. The resources available to conduct our review were limited and we had tight time scales in which to deliver. This was a challenge, especially given the fact that mixed methods reviews are a fairly recent development and the team conducting the review were applying the methodology for the first time. We had to make pragmatic decisions about how to make the review manageable within the resources available.

Although our review included international studies, it had a UK focus. We therefore included only qualitative studies from the UK as we considered the strengths of qualitative research to be in identifying the specific contextual factors shaping women's perspectives and experiences in the UK. All of our trials, however, were conducted in the US. This placed limits on the reach of the analysis. Ideally, for a fuller analysis of what works for whom and in what context it would have been useful to extend our inclusion criteria to qualitative studies conducted in other countries. A further useful source of information on reasons for why the interventions may not have achieved the anticipated outcomes would be to include trial authors insights as reported in, for example, the discussion sections of trial reports.

Although further worked examples of this approach are needed, overall the University of Sheffield team found that integrating qualitative and quantitative research within a mixed methods review framework offered several benefits. The approach has been well explained and the steps involved are in the main explicit and easy for others to pick up and use. There is flexibility in the approach as it is question-driven and tailored to accommodate the inclusion of a range of "quantitative" and "qualitative" studies and a range of synthesis methods within its different "sub-syntheses." The opportunity the method presents to create an explicit dialog between the qualitative and quantitative studies is a particularly attractive feature of the approach. As the other chapters in this book demonstrate, considerable effort has gone into developing methods for the synthesis of qualitative research over the past decade. In the context of trying to produce a more nuanced understanding of the effects of interventions, methods for integrating qualitative syntheses with effectiveness syntheses are much less well developed. The methods and approach described in this chapter are therefore an important contribution.

Conclusion

The mixed methods approach described in this chapter illustrates the value of drawing together the findings of a qualitative thematic synthesis with those of an effectiveness review. The framework for this approach is explicit and the review processes can be picked up with ease, as illustrated in the worked example. Identifying the recurring themes and issues that emerge from people's views and experiences of the policies and practices under review creates knowledge about the need, appropriateness, and acceptability of interventions. This approach increases understanding of why complex interventions may or may not work in different contexts, and can inform the development of future interventions and research.

References

Barnett-Page E, Thomas J. (2009) Methods for the synthesis of qualitative research: a critical review. *BMC Medical Research Methodology.* **9**: 59. doi: 10.1186/1471-2288-9-59.

Campbell F, Johnson M, Messina J, Guillaume L, Goyder E. (2010) Diet and/or physical activity -interventions for the prevention of excessive weight gain in women during pregnancy. A systematic review. 1–215. London: National Institute for Health and Clinical Excellence.

Chalmers, I. (2005) If evidence-informed policy works in practice, does it matter if it doesn't work in theory? *Evidence & Policy: A Journal of Research, Debate and Practice.* **1**(2): 227–242.

Creswell J. (2010) Mapping the developing landscape of mixed methods research. In: A Tashakkori, C Teddlie (Eds) *Mixed Methods Handbook* (2nd Edition). New York: Sage Publications.

Crossley N. (2004) Fat is a sociological issue: obesity rates in late modern, 'body conscious' societies. *Social Theory and Health.* **2**(3): 222–253.

Dixon-Woods M, Shaw RL, Agarwal S, Smith JA. (2004) The problem of appraising qualitative research. *Qual Saf Health Care.* **13**: 223225.

Dixon-Woods M, Bonas S, Booth A, Jones D, Miller T, Sutton A, Shaw R, Smith J, Young B. (2006a) How can systematic reviews incorporate qualitative research? A critical perspective. *Qualitative Research.* **6**: 27–44.

Dixon-Woods M, Cavers D, Agarwal S, Annandale E, Arthur A, Harvey J, Katbamna S, Olsen R, Smith L, Riley R, Sutton AJ. (2006b) Conducting a critical interpretative synthesis of the literature on access to healthcare by vulnerable groups. *BMC Med Res Methodol*. **6**: 35.

Egger M, Davey-Smith G, Altman D. (Eds) (2001) *Systematic Reviews in Health Care: Meta-analysis in Context*. London: BMJ Publishing.

Ely, JW, Osheroff, JA, Maviglia, SM, Rosenbaum, ME. (2007) Patient-care questions that physicians are unable to answer. *J Am Med Inform Assoc*. **14**: 407–414.

Fox P, Yamaguchi C. (1997) Body image change in pregnancy: a comparison of normal weight and overweight primigravidas. *Birth: Issues in Perinatal Care*. **24**(1): 35–40.

Greenhalgh T, Robert G, Macfarlane F, Bate P, Kyriakidou O, Peacock R. (2005) Storylines of research in diffusion of innovation: a meta-narrative approach to systematic review. *Social Science & Medicine*. **61**(2): 417–30.

Gross H, Bee P. (2004) Perceptions of effective advice in pregnancy - The case of activity. *Clinical Effectiveness in Nursing*. **8**: 161–169.

Guba, EG. (1987). What have we learned about naturalistic evaluation? *Evaluation Practice*. **8**(1): 23–42.

Harden A, Thomas J. (2005) Methodological issues in combining diverse study types in systematic reviews. *International Journal of Social Research Methods*. **8**: 257–271.

Harden A, Thomas J. (2010) Mixed methods and systematic reviews: examples and emerging issues. In A Tashakkori, C Teddlie (Eds) *Mixed Methods Handbook* (2nd Edition). New York: Sage Publications.

Higgins JPT, Green S. (Eds). (2009) *Cochrane Handbook for Systematic Reviews of Interventions* Version 5.0.2 [updated September 2009]. The Cochrane Collaboration. Available from www.cochrane-handbook.org [accessed 7 June 2011].

Kanagalingam MG, Forouhi NG, Greer IA, Sattar N. (2005) Changing in booking body mass over a decade: retrospective analysis from a Glasgow maternity hospital. *BJOG*. **112**: 1431–1433.

Lewis, G. (Ed). (2007) The Confidential Enquiry into Maternal and Child Health (CEMACH). Saving Mothers' Lives: Reviewing Maternal Deaths to Make Motherhood Safer - 2003–2005. The Seventh Report on Confidential Enquiries into Maternal Deaths in the United Kingdom. London: CEMACH.

Lipsey M, Wilson D. (2001) *Practical Meta-analysis*. Thousand Oaks, California, Sage.

National Institute for health and Clinical Excellence (2006) Public Health Guidance: Development Process and Methods. London: National Institute for Health and Clinical Excellence. (http://www.nice.org.uk/media/2FB/53/PHMethodsManual110509.pdf [accessed 7 June 2011])

Noblit GW, Hare RD. (1988) *Meta-Ethnography: Synthesizing Qualitative Studies*. Newbury Park, Sage.

Noyes J, Popay J, Pearson A, Hannes H, Booth A. (2008) Qualitative research and Cochrane reviews. In JPT Higgins and S Green (Eds) *Cochrane Handbook of Systematic Reviews of Interventions*. Chap 20. John Wiley & Sons, Chichester.

Oliver S, Harden A, Rees R, Shepherd J, Brunton G, Garcia J, Oakley A. (2005) An emerging framework for integrating different types of evidence in systematic reviews for public policy. *Evaluation*. **11**: 428–66.

Roberts A, Noyes J. (2009) Contraception and women over 40 years of age: mixed-method systematic review. *Journal of Advanced Nursing*. **65**(6): 1155–1170. doi: 10.1111/j.1365-2648.2009.04976.x.

Sheiner E, Levy A, Menes TS, Silverberg D, Katz M, Mazor M. (2004) Maternal obesity as an independent risk factor for caesarean delivery. *Paediatric and Perinatal Epidemiology.* **18**(3): 196–201.

Strauss AL, Corbin J. (1998) *Basics of Qualitative Research: Techniques and Procedures for Developing Grounded Theory.* Thousand Oaks, CA: Sage.

Thomas J, Brunton J, Graziosi S. (2010) EPPI-Reviewer 4.0: software for research synthesis. EPPI-Centre Software. Social Science Research Unit, Institute of Education, London.

Thomas J, Harden A, Oakley A, Oliver S, Sutcliffe K, Rees R, Brunton G, Kavanagh J. (2004) Integrating qualitative research with trials in systematic reviews: an example from public health. *British Medical Journal.* **328**: 1010–12.

Thomas J, Harden A. (2008) Methods for the thematic synthesis of qualitative research in systematic reviews *BMC Medical Research Methodology.* **8**: 45.

Warin M, Turner K, Moore V, Davies M. (2008) Bodies, mothers and identities: rethinking obesity and the BMI. *Sociology of Health and Illness.* **30**(1): 97–111.

Warriner S. (2000) Women's views on being weighed during pregnancy. *BR J Midwifery.* **8**(10): 620–623.

Chapter 7 Bayesian approaches to the synthesis of qualitative and quantitative research findings

Jamie L. Crandell, PhD[1], Corrine I. Voils, PhD[2], and Margarete Sandelowski, PhD, RN[3]

[1]University of North Carolina at Chapel Hill, NC, USA

[2]Durham Veterans Affairs Medical Center and Duke University Medical Center, Durham, NC, USA

[3]University of North Carolina at Chapel Hill, Chapel Hill, NC, USA

The Bayesian statistical framework naturally combines information from different sources, making it especially applicable to mixed research synthesis. We illustrate three different Bayesian approaches to the synthesis of qualitative and quantitative research findings to address the research question "Which factors are associated with HIV antiretroviral medication adherence?" Although all three approaches were designed to incorporate information from both types of studies, they use this information in different ways. The assumptions, advantages, and disadvantages of each approach are discussed.

Introduction

Over the last decade, there has been a surge of interest in mixed research synthesis, or studies that entail the integration of both qualitative and quantitative findings. Among the array of methods proposed are Bayesian approaches (Pope *et al.* 2007). Bayesian methods tend to be more computationally intensive than classical statistical methods, so technological advances over the past couple of decades have accelerated the use and development of these approaches in meta-analysis (Sutton & Abrams 2001). In this chapter, we feature three Bayesian approaches to synthesizing qualitative and quantitative research findings: an approach described by Roberts *et al.* (2002) and approaches described in two of our own papers (Voils *et al.* 2009 and Crandell *et al.* in press).

Synthesizing Qualitative Research: Choosing the Right Approach, First Edition.
Edited by Karin Hannes and Craig Lockwood.
© 2012 John Wiley & Sons, Ltd. Published 2012 by John Wiley & Sons, Ltd.

An overview of the Bayesian framework

The earliest forms of formal research synthesis developed around classical (frequentist) statistical methods, with a recent shift towards incorporation of Bayesian techniques. One strength of the Bayesian statistical framework is its inherent ability to synthesize information from multiple sources, thereby making it especially useful for integrating findings from methodologically diverse studies. In a widely-used textbook on Bayesian analysis, Gelman *et al.* (2004, p. 3) described the Bayesian approach as a set of "practical methods for using probability models for quantities which we observe and for quantities about which we wish to learn." The phrase "quantities which we observe" refers to collected data, while "quantities about which we wish to learn" refers to model parameters (i.e., the quantities the researcher is trying to estimate about the population – often means, effect sizes, probabilities, or odds ratios). At its foundation, Bayesian inference involves building probability models for both the observed data and the model parameters. This is in contrast to frequentist statistical methods in which probability models are used for observed data but never for model parameters.

This is a difficult concept, but may be made simpler through an example. Consider the p-value, a widely used probability in frequentist approaches, which can be loosely interpreted as "the probability that we would obtain data similar to what we observed if the null hypothesis were really true." If the p-value is low (usually $<.05$), we reject the null hypothesis, concluding our data would have been very unlikely if it were true. The complicated interpretation of the p-value is based on the frequentist conceptualization of probability – that probability can only be used to express uncertainty about events that contain innate randomness (in this case, the sampling process, or the measurement process), not uncertainty about population quantities (parameters) that are unknown. In the frequentist paradigm, declaring, for example, "the probability that the null hypothesis is true" is not valid because the truth of the null hypothesis is fixed (not random), whether we know it or not.

In reality, humans make probability statements about processes not subject to sampling or measurement error quite often (e.g., the probability the check cleared the bank today, or the probability the bus is already waiting at the stop). In general conversation, people use probability in the Bayesian way to quantify uncertainty about the situation. Bayesian thinking expands the scope of frequentist thinking by allowing assignment probabilities not just to the data, but to our hypotheses (if we have them) or to other statements about the population. In general, Bayesian analysis is usually less focused on hypothesis-testing than frequentist analysis, but its flexible definition of probability allows us to let population parameters follow a statistical distribution, where the variability in the distribution represents our uncertainty about those parameters.

A Bayesian analysis usually proceeds in three steps: 1) quantifying our uncertainty about the population parameters (unknown quantities about the population – e.g., means, variances, odds, ratios, etc.) by writing a probability distribution for these parameters; 2) examining the relationship between the observed data and these unknown parameters; and 3) refining our initial uncertainty about the parameters based on the data. The three steps follow in more detail.

Step 1. The prior distribution

The most widely exploited advantage of Bayesian analysis is the ability to incorporate prior (i.e., before data collection) information about the distribution of each parameter of interest. In classical analysis, the information about the parameter is limited to that provided by the observed data. In Bayesian analysis, before the data are even collected, researchers can provide an educated estimate of the statistical distribution of the parameter. This distribution represents the researchers' uncertainty about the parameter's value. If researchers are quite uncertain about the value, they will create a prior distribution that allows a wide range of values with approximately equal probability (called a *flat* or *non-informative* prior distribution). If they already have data or theory suggesting a parameter should fall in a narrow range, then the prior distribution will be *informative*, allowing only a narrow range with high probability and possibly having one or more values that are "most likely."

As a statistical distribution, the prior distribution is simply a mathematical function of the model parameters. When the prior distribution is evaluated at specific values of the parameters, the result is a number, with a higher number indicating the current values are a priori more likely to be the true population values.

Step 2. The likelihood

Like the prior, the likelihood is also a statistical distribution. Whereas the prior distribution represents uncertainty about the parameters, the likelihood represents the relative likelihood of different values of parameters leading to the observed data. The likelihood is written as a function of the observed data (numbers) and the unknown parameters whose prior distribution has already been specified.

As is the case for the prior, when the likelihood is evaluated at specific values of the model parameters, the result is simply a number, and a higher value of the likelihood indicates that the observed data are more likely to occur if those specific parameter values are the true population values.

Step 3. The posterior distribution

The posterior distribution is a statistical distribution summarizing the information contained in the prior distribution and the likelihood about the parameters. The posterior distribution is created using Bayes' rule:

$$P(\text{parameters} \mid \text{data}) = \frac{P(\text{data} \mid \text{parameters})\, P(\text{parameters})}{P(\text{data})}$$

$$= \frac{\text{likelihood} \times \text{prior}}{P(\text{data})}$$

The distribution of the parameters alone – P(parameters) – is the prior distribution. The distribution of the data conditional on the parameters – P(data | parameters) – is the likelihood. The distribution of the parameters conditional on the observed data – P(parameters | data) – is the posterior distribution. P(data) is a numerical constant, which is designated here as 1/C. The following equation relates the posterior distribution to the likelihood and the prior:

$$\text{posterior distribution} = C \times \text{likelihood} \times \text{prior}$$

The value of C is generally irrelevant because the posterior distribution indicates the relative probability of different values of the parameters being correct given the observed data; dividing the entire distribution by a constant does not change the relative probability of two different parameter values. There are methods for deriving the value of C, but they are outside the scope of this chapter.

It is common to summarize what has been learned about the parameters from the observed data with a measure of central tendency (e.g., mean, median, or mode) of the posterior distribution and a credible interval. A credible interval is the Bayesian analog to a confidence interval, so a 95% credible interval will describe a range of values from the posterior distribution in which the parameter lies with 95% probability.

Applying Bayesian methods to mixed research synthesis

The utility of the Bayesian approach in research synthesis stems from its relaxed definition of probability and its reliance on combining distributions. Every synthesis requires a slightly different approach, tailored to the subject matter and the available evidence, and Bayesian methods are more amenable than frequentist methods to slight alterations.

A research synthesis conducted in a Bayesian framework begins the same way as a research synthesis in any other framework with the formulation of research questions, gathering of research reports, extraction of information from these reports, and selection of extracted data for synthesis. The data extracted will be driven by the type of analysis that is planned. The three examples featured here illustrate how Bayesian methods may be used in various ways to synthesize qualitative and quantitative findings.

The purpose of the parent study from which the analyses in this chapter are derived was to develop methods to synthesize qualitative and quantitative research findings. The domains of literature used were qualitative, quantitative observational, and intervention studies of (a) stigma and of (b) antiretroviral medication adherence in HIV-positive persons. Over the five-year course of the study, we searched 40 databases across the health, behavioral, and social sciences with variants of key search terms; in the case of antiretroviral medication adherence studies, these terms included adherence, compliance, antiretroviral, HAART, HIV/AIDS, and the like. Each project within the parent study drew from different parts of the total collection of reports of studies, numbering about 250. The reports featured here were selected as relevant to using and further developing Bayesian approaches to synthesis. (Further information on search and retrieval procedures is available from the authors on request.) The research question asked of this set of reports for the Bayesian analyses was: "Which factors are (positively or negatively) associated with antiretroviral medication adherence?"

We present three Bayesian approaches for synthesizing qualitative and quantitative research findings (hereafter referred to as *data*) to answer this research question. In the first approach, described by Voils *et al.* (2009), the defining feature is the conversion of qualitative data into numbers so that these qualitative data could be used together with the quantitative data to calculate the likelihood. Using a popular term in the mixed methods research literature (Tashakkori & Teddlie 2003), we refer to it here simply as the "quantitizing" approach. In the second approach, described by Crandell *et al.* (in press), the defining feature is coding the presence/absence of themes in both qualitative and quantitative reports so that these data can be used together to create the likelihood. Using another popular term in the mixed methods literature, we refer to it here simply as the "qualitizing" approach. In the third approach, described by Roberts *et al.* (2002), the defining feature is using data from the qualitative reports to create the prior distributions, which are then updated with data from the quantitative reports. We refer to it here simply as the "qualitative-as-prior" approach.

The quantitizing approach

The defining feature of the quantitizing approach (Voils *et al.* 2009) is the conversion of verbal counts in qualitative studies into numbers for inclusion in the likelihood along with the data from quantitative studies. This approach is best suited for low-inference, or minimally interpreted, qualitative descriptive findings, not for highly interpreted findings in the form of grounded theories, phenomenologies, and the like (Sandelowski & Barroso 2007). This approach is designed to compute the degree of support in empirical studies for a single hypothesized relationship between two variables. Voils *et al.* (2009) hypothesized that decreased adherence would be associated with more complex medication regimens.

As stated in Voils *et al* (2009, p. 227), "regimen complexity is a broad category of factors commonly appearing in systematic reviews of research on antiretroviral adherence and consisting of an array of diverse factors." Because this variability among studies is common in many research areas, research synthesis is often of findings addressing similar, but not identical, topics. In this synthesis, "we included in the category of 'medication regimen complexity' any finding addressing dosing frequency, size of pills, timing of medications, availability of medication refills, medication side effects, ease or difficulty of incorporation of pill-taking into daily routine, dietary requirements of drugs, and regimen changes" (Voils *et al.* 2009, p. 228). Regimen complexity was addressed in 21 reports: 11 qualitative and 10 quantitative.

For example, a qualitative report might contain the statement that "several participants reported that using reminder devices such as timers improved their adherence to an antiretroviral regimen," whereas a quantitative report might contain the statement that "out of 50 respondents, 11 responded that using reminder devices such as timers improved their adherence to an antiretroviral regimen." Both of these findings are informative, but the number (11 out of 50) cannot be directly synthesized with the word *several*. Accordingly, Chang *et al.* (2009) developed a method for the conversion of such verbal counts in qualitative reports to plausible numbers of participants associated with findings. Using this method, which involves using regression equations to predict what is commonly interpreted by a given word in the context of sample size, if the qualitative study in the example above had 25 participants, *several* would denote 2–13 participants. A likelihood is then constructed that describes the range for each of the qualitative studies, assuming that every number in the range is equally likely. A separate likelihood is constructed that describes the quantitative studies, in which the findings are not ranges of estimated numbers of participants, but actual observed numbers of participants. The qualitative studies and quantitative studies were then synthesized separately. Because qualitative and quantitative studies are typically conceived as methodologically different, all of the qualitative studies could be seen as estimating one probability and all of the quantitative studies as estimating another probability. If the posterior distributions turn out to be different, this may be an indication that the two study types are not estimating the same probability and, arguably, that the distributions should not be combined.

The quantitizing approach: prior distribution

Voils *et al.* (2009) wanted to allow the qualitative and quantitative findings to provide the weight of evidence for the posterior distribution (i.e., desired no prior information) and therefore used a uniform prior distribution, which is non-informative, defining the same prior probability for every possible scenario.

The quantitizing approach: data extraction and likelihood

Construction of the likelihood involved obtaining counts of participants expressing the association between regimen complexity and non-adherence from both qualitative and quantitative reports. From the quantitative reports, we used unadjusted results (proportions, probabilities, percentages, or relative risk) to compute the number of participants associated with each finding. Four reports were excluded: two for which the outcome was mean adherence with no way to count the number of subjects expressing an association, and two others that provided only covariate-adjusted adherence rates. (Unadjusted rates were not available from the authors.) After these exclusions, it was possible to count the number of participants supporting the hypothesis in six of the quantitative reports (Table 7.1). In five of the six reports, the variable addressing regimen complexity was regimen type (HAART [highly active anti-retroviral therapy] versus pre-HAART, or combination therapy versus monotherapy); in one study, the variable was having too many pills xto take. Table 7.1 shows the number of subjects supporting the relationship between regimen complexity and non-adherence from both the qualitative and quantitative reports.

The quantitizing approach: constructing the posterior distribution

For each type of data (qualitative and quantitative) the likelihood was combined with the prior distribution to generate posterior distributions using Mathematica software (Wolfram 1996). A complete exposition of the mathematical methods used is available in the original manuscript (Voils *et al.* 2009) and requires in-depth mathematical understanding of statistical distributions and random effects models (see, for example, the chapter on hierarchical models in Gelman *et al.* 2004). A brief overview of the statistical model is given here.

Table 7.1 Findings synthesized in the quantitizing approach. Adapted from Voils *et al.* 2009 with permission from the Royal Society of Medicine Press, London.

	Report	Total study N	Number reporting more complex regimen associated with lower adherence*
Qualitative	Abel & Painter 2003	6	2 to 6
	Gant & Welch 2004	30	3 to 15
	Misener & Sowell 1998	22	6 to 22
	Powell-Cope *et al.* 2003	24	13 to 24
	Remien *et al.* 2003	110	56 to 110
	Richter *et al.* 2002	33	2 to 33
	Roberts & Mann 2000	20	15 to 20
	Schrimshaw *et al.* 2005	158	100 to 142
	Siegel & Gorey 1997	71	15 to 71
	Siegel *et al.* 2001	51	11 to 51
	Wood *et al.* 2004	36	2 to 36
Quantitative	Durante *et al.* 2003	48	12
	Phillips *et al.* 2005	125	21
	Schuman *et al.* 2001	326	57
	Stone *et al.* 2001	186	59
	Wilson *et al.* 2002	562	136
	Wilson *et al.* 2001	132	25

*For qualitative reports, estimated ranges are given. For quantitative reports, numbers are extracted from the reports directly.

Each participant in one of the chosen reports (qualitative or quantitative) can be thought of as an independent entity with probability p of supporting the link between regimen complexity and non-adherence. If it can be assumed that p is the same for every study, then the data from all participants would follow a binomial likelihood. The authors found evidence of heterogeneity among the quantitative studies (i.e., they did not all have the same underlying p), suggesting that a fixed effects model (i.e., a single value of p) is inappropriate. Therefore, they used the beta-binomial random effects model, which allows p to vary across studies according to the beta distribution (Kleinman 1973). Model parameters were estimated using the modified Gauss–Newton method (Hartley 1961).

The quantitizing approach: results
The resulting posterior probabilities from the qualitative and quantitative studies are shown in Figure 7.1. The posterior mode for the probability of adherence in the qualitative studies was 0.588 (95% credible interval

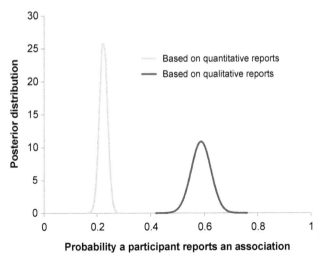

Figure 7.1 Posterior distributions for the quantitizing method. Adapted from Voils *et al.* 2009 with permission from the Royal Society of Medicine Press, London.

0.519, 0.663). For the quantitative studies, the posterior mode for the probability of association was 0.224 (0.203, 0.245).

The point estimates for the qualitative and quantitative studies were vastly different, so it is possible that each set of findings is estimating a different mean probability (i.e., there is heterogeneity between study types for this research question). This may be due to the nature of the individual studies, the method for converting verbal counts in qualitative reports (i.e., over-estimating the number of participants associated with a finding), or an inherent methodological difference between qualitative and quantitative studies. If the posterior distributions for the two study types were more similar, they could be mathematically combined to produce a single posterior distribution. Due to the observed heterogeneity, the authors chose not to combine them. Mathematically, any two distributions can be combined, so the degree of overlap required before combining is at the discretion of the researcher, necessitating careful consideration of the credible intervals and histograms of the posterior distributions. A researcher who desires a Bayesian significance test for whether two distributions share the same mean/mode/median can refer to Chapter 6 in Gelman *et al.* (2004), which discusses Bayesian hypothesis testing

Whereas this quantitizing approach addressed only the association between one factor (regimen complexity) and adherence, the next two Bayesian approaches are able to address multiple factors simultaneously. Reading the qualitative and quantitative reports yielded four factors that were most often mentioned as related to adherence: side effects/feeling ill, having or living with children, negative feelings, and the presence of a positive social network. We examine these four factors in the next two approaches.

The qualitizing approach

This Bayesian approach, exemplified in the analysis described by Crandell *et al.* (in press), is focused also on extracting themes from qualitative reports, but not on inferring plausible ranges of numerical values. Rather, given a set of potential associations, each report (qualitative and quantitative) is categorized according to whether it supports an association. An advantage of this approach is that statistical methods for missing data can be applied, which is important because reports in any research synthesis project will never address all of the same possible associations.

The qualitizing approach: prior distribution

As in the quantitizing approach, this approach (Crandell *et al.* in press) allows evidence from the qualitative and quantitative studies to provide the weight of evidence in the posterior distribution. In order to accomplish this, a normal prior distribution with a very large variance was chosen, essentially behaving as a non-informative prior.

The qualitizing approach: data extraction and likelihood

Crandell *et al.* (in press) first created a data matrix (Table 7.2) summarizing the findings of all of the reports addressing at least one of the selected factors, with each column corresponding to one factor and each row to a single report. Initially, the intent was to code the relationship with adherence dichotomously: either there is a relationship, or there is not. The authors found, however, a need to denote the direction of the association because some factors (i.e., side effects/ feeling ill and having children) were reported as being a barrier to adherence in some reports and a facilitator of adherence in others. This variation must not be lost in the synthesis. Thus, entries were made in the matrix whenever the factor was reported as promoting adherence (1), having no effect on adherence (0.5), or promoting non-adherence (0). Cells were left blank if the relationship was not addressed at all. The criterion for an association in the quantitative reports was a statistically significant finding supporting the relationship (at a significance level of .05); in the qualitative reports, it was a statement by the report's author(s) supporting the relationship (regardless of how many participants stated the relationship, but at least one). Non-significant findings or statements indicating the absence of a relationship were coded as 0.5. One requirement of

Table 7.2 Data and results for the qualitizing approach

		Side effects/feeling ill	Having or living with children	Negative feelings	Positive social network
Qualitative	Abel & Painter 2003	0		0	
	Edwards 2006				1
	Gant & Welch 2004		1		1
	Misener & Sowell 1998	0			0.5
	Powell-Cope et al. 2003	0	0	0	1
	Richter et al. 2002	1			
	Roberts & Mann 2000	0	0		
	Schrimshaw et al. 2005	0			
	Siegel & Gorey 1997	0			
	Siegel et al. 2001	0			
	Wood et al. 2004	0	1		1
Quantitative	Douglass et al. 2003	0			1
	Durante et al. 2003				1
	Howard et al. 2002	0.5	0.5		
	Kalichman et al. 2001		1	0	
	Liu et al. 2006				0.5
	Mostashari et al. 1998				1
	Murphy et al. 2002				0.5
	Phillips et al. 2005			0	
	Sowell et al. 2001	0.5			
	Stone et al. 2001			0.5	
	Wilson et al. 2002				0.5
Posterior mean and 95% credible interval		.84 (.75, .95)	.63 (.41, .84)	.21 (.08, .34)	.19 (.09, .31)

this method is variability across studies; if the same conclusion is drawn about a single factor in all studies, this approach is not applicable because it relies on the estimation of a variance between studies.

The qualitizing approach: constructing the posterior distribution

Table 7.2 has a large proportion of empty cells. As is usually the case in research synthesis studies, not every factor was mentioned in every report.

Because the dataset had only a small number of observed cells, Crandell *et al.* (in press) focused their attention on the exploration of standard methods for dealing with missing data. The most straightforward approach would have been a complete case analysis, including only reports that addressed all of the variables (i.e., use only "complete" observations). There were no reports that met that criterion, which is likely to be the case in most applications. Crandell *et al.* also demonstrate a complete-case method for analyzing each factor separately, in which the small sample size yields very wide confidence intervals and hard-to-interpret results.

Whenever excessive loss of data makes it unacceptable to analyze only complete observations, several methods can be employed (Little & Rubin 2002). The most widely used of these methods rely on Bayesian approaches to impute the values of the missing data, then analyze the data as if they were complete. The Bayesian data augmentation method used (Gelman 2004) is relatively straightforward to implement and is appropriate for any amount of missing data. This method assumes that each row in the table, if completely observed, could be considered a random vector drawn from some type of multivariate statistical distribution. In reality, only a few elements from each vector are observed, and all others are unobserved (missing). The data augmentation procedure involves using the observed data to estimate the unknown parameters of the multivariate distribution, then drawing from the distribution to estimate the missing values themselves. The estimated missing values are then used to fill in the empty cells in the dataset, and the parameters of the underlying statistical distribution are re-estimated. This procedure is repeated until a large number of estimates have been obtained, and the large number of estimates is then summarized to describe the multivariate distribution from which each row was drawn.

The model assumes that each column (i.e., factor) had its own underlying mean around which the values (observed and unobserved) were centered. Gibbs sampling is a common method for drawing samples from a posterior distribution, and a large number is drawn in order to provide the most accurate summary of the posterior. After verifying that the sampling process had converged, the Gibbs Sampler drew 18 000 estimates from the underlying distribution, which can be considered as 18 000 random draws from the posterior distribution of the four column means. (See Gelman *et al.* 2004 for an in-depth discussion of Gibbs sampling.)

The qualitizing approach: results

Point estimates and credible intervals were constructed by summarizing the 18 000 samples. The point estimate of each mean is the average over all the samples, and can be used to describe the evidence for a relationship between each factor and adherence/non-adherence. A 95% credible interval for each estimate was simply the 2.5th and 97.5th percentiles of the 18 000 samples, because the samples from the posterior distribution fell in that range 95% of the time.

The point estimates and 95% credible intervals for the means are provided at the bottom of Table 7.2. A value of zero in the table indicates that a factor is associated with non-adherence to the regimen, a value of .5 means there is no association between the factor and adherence, and a value of 1 means that a factor is associated with adherence. Therefore, if a confidence interval contains .5, there is not enough evidence to categorically state an association with either adherence or non-adherence. If the interval is below .5, then the factor is associated with non-adherence; if the interval is above .5, then the factor is associated with adherence. As shown in Table 7.2, the results indicate that a positive social network promotes adherence, having children has an undetermined effect on adherence, and side effects/feeling ill and negative feelings promote non-adherence.

Another advantage of this approach is that the samples from the posterior distribution can be used to compare the relative ranking of the importance of each factor. For example, the authors computed the probability that side effects/feeling ill was more promoting of non-adherence than negative feelings. To do this, they computed the percentage of samples in which the estimated mean for side effects/feeling ill was lower than that for negative feelings. This occurred in 7889 samples, or 44% of the time. The data therefore support a 44% chance that side effects/feeling ill is more detrimental to adherence than negative feelings.

This is a type of Bayesian hypothesis testing. With a 44% chance that side effects/feeling ill is more detrimental, there is a 56% chance that negative feelings are more detrimental. The posterior probability of 44% is not enough evidence to conclude that one factor is more or less important than the other.

The qualitative-as-prior approach

Roberts *et al.* (2002) and Lilford and Braunholtz (2003) proposed using qualitative data to create an informative prior distribution, which is then updated with the likelihood derived from the results from the quantitative studies. Roberts *et al.* (2002) applied this approach to a study of factors contributing to the uptake of immunization. In this section, we illustrate their method by using it to identify factors associated with adherence/non-adherence to an antiretroviral medication regimen.

In this approach, we used the same four factors studied in the qualitizing approach. Yet, there were two main differences at the outset. The first difference was that we extracted odds ratios (and their variances) from the quantitative reports. The second difference was the way that the qualitative findings were converted into numerical values for analysis. Although we were able to account for the ambiguity of a factor being associated with adherence sometimes and non-adherence at other times in the qualitizing approach, allowing for more than one direction of association is incompatible with the method Roberts *et al.* (2002) proposed. Consequently, for each association between a factor and adherence, we had to indicate the direction of association (i.e., whether the factor promotes or hinders adherence) and then code each study accordingly. Each hypothesis about the direction of influence is shown at the top of Table 7.3.

The qualitative-as-prior approach: prior distribution

For each of the four hypothesized relationships, we used the qualitative reports to generate a prior probability. These probabilities were the proportion of the qualitative reports indicating the finding to be true. For example, 8 out of 11 qualitative reports indicated that side effects diminished adherence, yielding a prior probability of $8/11 = 73\%$. The prior probabilities for the remaining three factors are shown in Table 7.3. Roberts *et al.* (2002) also indicated that a panel of experts can be used to state prior probabilities in light of personal experience and the qualitative evidence.

The qualitative-as-prior approach: data extraction and likelihood

From the quantitative reports, we extracted odds ratios indicating the strength of the relationship between each of the hypotheses. These odds ratios are given in Table 7.3. Odds ratios greater than 1 indicate a relationship between the factor and adherence, and odds ratios less than 1 indicate a relationship between the factor and non-adherence. The variance of the log-odds, which is required for computation, is given in parentheses.

The prior probabilities from the qualitative reports were used to construct the prior distributions for the pooled odds ratios. For example, the odds ratio between side effects and adherence was given an a priori 73% chance of being

Table 7.3 Data and results for the qualitative-as-prior approach

	Side effects/ feeling ill decreases adherence	Having or living with children improves adherence	Negative feelings decrease adherence	Positive social network improves adherence
Qualitative: Presence of theme?				
Abel & Painter 2003	yes	no	yes	no
Edwards 2006	no	no	no	yes
Gant & Welch 2004	yes	yes	no	yes
Misener & Sowell 1998	yes	no	no	no
Powell-Cope et al. 2003	yes	no	yes	yes
Richter et al. 2002	no	no	no	no
Roberts & Mann 2000	yes	no	no	no
Schrimshaw et al. 2005	yes	no	no	no
Siegel & Gorey 1997	yes	no	no	no
Siegel et al. 2001	yes	no	no	no
Wood et al. 2004	no	yes	no	yes
Prior probabilities from qualitative reports	73%	18%	18%	36%
Quantitative: Odds ratio and variance of the log-odds ratio				
Douglass et al. 2003	0.526 (0.116)			3.014 (0.123)
Durante et al. 2003				2.536 (0.246)
Howard et al. 2002	0.926 (0.083)	0.928 (0.087)		
Kalichman et al. 2001		2.550 (0.382)	0.280 (0.248)	1.056 (0.185)
Liu et al. 2006				
Mostashari et al. 1998				3.900 (0.274)
Murphy et al. 2002				1.141 (0.394)
Phillips et al. 2005			0.403 (0.123)	
Sowell et al. 2001	1.388 (0.042)			
Stone et al. 2001			0.930 (0.064)	
Wilson et al. 2002				1.373 (0.038)
Posterior probabilities after synthesis	46%	71%	99.6%	99.98%

less than 1. The odds ratio between having children and adherence was given an a priori 18% chance of being greater than 1.

The qualitative-as-prior approach: constructing the posterior distribution

The prior evidence was updated with the data from the quantitative reports; the posterior probability is given in the last row of Table 7.3. Our calculations were performed according to the methods described in Jones *et al.* (2005, pers. comm.). Briefly, the prior distribution of the underlying log-odds ratio was assumed to be normal with variance of .16 (chosen by us to yield a fairly informative prior distribution, as no value was recommended in Jones *et al.* (2005, pers. comm.). The prior mean was chosen so that the log-odds ratio had the stated prior probability of being greater than 1 (for factors hypothesized to improve adherence) or less than 1 (for factors hypothesized to decrease adherence). The likelihood was written as that for a fixed-effects model, assuming each observed log-odds ratio to be drawn from a distribution with the same underlying mean. The prior and likelihood were combined to generate a posterior distribution for the mean log-odds ratio. The posterior probability given is the posterior probability that the mean log odds-ratio was greater than 1 (for factors hypothesized to improve adherence) or less than 1 (for factors hypothesized to decrease adherence).

The qualitative-as-prior approach: results

In all cases, the posterior probability of the hypothesis was quite different from the prior probability, indicating the quantitative evidence was very strong, outweighing the qualitative evidence. For example, a positive social network was mentioned in only 3 of the 11 qualitative reports as promoting adherence, but the weight of the quantitative evidence increased this probability dramatically.

Discussion of the three approaches

Although Bayesian synthesis has been advanced as a way to incorporate prior information into a synthesis (Dixon-Woods *et al.* 2004; Pope *et al.* 2007), the Bayesian paradigm may also be used to overcome several limitations of the frequentist approach to research synthesis. The Bayesian paradigm may be used to synthesize ranges of numbers rather than point estimates (quantitizing approach), to borrow information across studies to reduce uncertainty (qualitizing approach), or to incorporate prior information into a quantitative synthesis (qualitative-as-prior approach).

Table 7.4 summarizes a comparison among the three applied approaches. In the quantitizing approach, qualitative findings are translated into plausible

Table 7.4 Comparison of three Bayesian approaches

	Quantitizing approach	Qualitizing approach	Qualitative-as-prior approach
Number of associations/hypotheses examined simultaneously	Examines evidence for a single association between two variables	Examines evidence for multiple associations based on a collection of reports, all of which may not address each association	Examines evidence for multiple hypotheses based on a collection of reports, all of which may not address each hypothesis
Form of qualitative data	Converts verbal counts into numerical ranges	Codes qualitative reports on support or lack thereof for associations (i.e., whether a factor is associated with the outcome positively, negatively, or not at all) based on thematic statements	Codes qualitative reports on support or lack thereof (i.e., yes or no) for hypothesized relationship based on thematic statements
Form of quantitative data	Uses quantitative data in the form of number of participants supporting the finding and total sample size	Codes quantitative reports on support or lack thereof for associations (based on, e.g., statistical significance or effect size)	Uses quantitative data in the form of odds ratios and variances
How qualitative and quantitative data are synthesized	Qualitative and quantitative data converted into same form (numerical counts) for inclusion in the likelihood	Qualitative and quantitative data converted into same form (categorical variable representing support for associations) for inclusion in the likelihood	Qualitative data are used to construct the prior; quantitative data are used to construct the likelihood

numerical values based on the language used by the author. The utility of the Bayesian framework is the ability to synthesize the ranges of numbers from the qualitative reports with the counts/proportions from the quantitative reports. This approach is successful in its inclusion of quantitative data in its most detailed form. A limitation is the newly developed methodology for the conversion of qualitative data into counts of participants. For example, the current method yields a range of counts in which the true value is assumed to lie, with equal probability of taking any value. In fact, there are probably numbers in the range that are more likely to be the true value than others, and a non-uniform distribution might be more appropriate. Further development of this methodology will increase the utility of this approach.

The qualitizing approach is focused not on converting verbal counts from qualitative reports, but rather determining whether – given a set of hypotheses – each qualitative and quantitative report: (a) provides evidence for a positive association; (b) provides evidence for a negative association; (c) provides evidence against any association; or (d) does not address the association.

Reports in the first three categories provide evidence about the existence and direction of an association; reports in the fourth category provide no information and can therefore be thought of as missing data. Statistical methods for missing data can be applied to conduct the synthesis. A Bayesian data augmentation algorithm can be used to allow for dependence among hypotheses. A defining feature of this method is its treatment of every report, whether qualitative or quantitative, as a single case in a dataset. This approach provides a summary of the literature but does not account for the relative weight of the evidence in individual studies. This approach could be expanded to retain its qualitizing nature while including weights (e.g., sample size) so that studies do not contribute equally to the conclusions.

Both the quantitizing and qualitizing approaches exploit the flexibility of Bayesian computation while reconciling the formats of qualitative and quantitative data so that they can be directly combined using non-informative prior distributions. The qualitative-as-prior approach does not entail the use of both qualitative and quantitative data in the likelihood, but rather the use of qualitative data to create an informative prior distribution, which is then updated with the likelihood describing the results from the quantitative reports. Thus it does not share the limitations of the other two approaches. Rather, its main limitation is that it is unclear how to be certain that both types of evidence contribute adequately to the conclusions. The choice of prior distribution in the qualitative-as-prior approach dictates the weight assigned to the body of qualitative evidence; a small variance gives more weight to the prior probability (i.e., qualitative studies) and a large variance gives more weight to the data (i.e., quantitative studies). Investigation of the nature of the effects of the prior variance should be undertaken by researchers using this method.

The qualitizing and qualitative-as-prior approaches were designed to test a set of associations/hypotheses simultaneously, and compare the weight of evidence for each of them, whereas the quantitizing approach was designed to examine only one association at a time, quantifying the strength of that association in detail. The quantitizing method might be less suitable than the others for comparing many factors' relationships with an outcome.

The qualitizing and qualitative-as-prior approach were used to synthesize essentially the same reports about whether adherence is related to side effects/ feeling ill, negative feelings, and the presence of a positive social network. The conclusions about negative feelings and positive social network were the same for both approaches (i.e., the association with adherence was strong). Yet, the qualitiative-as-prior approach did not yield strong evidence for an association between side effects/feeling ill and adherence whereas the qualitizing approach did find this evidence. For this particular factor, the weight of evidence from the literature seems to come from the qualitative studies (see Tables 7.2 and 7.3). The qualitative-as-prior approach had a 73% prior probability of an association, which was based entirely on the qualitative studies, but this probability was reduced to a 46% posterior probability once the quantitative evidence was considered. In the qualitizing approach, each report's finding inherently carries equal weight, so these qualitative studies were accounted for differently, producing a different result.

All three approaches yield results in a slightly different form. The quantitizing approach, which synthesizes at the subject level, yields a distribution for the probability of an association in a single subject, which can be reported as a probability and a credible interval for that probability. The qualitizing approach also yields a probability and credible interval for each association of interest, but this is the probability of an association on the report level. The qualitative-as-prior approach gives a probability that the pooled odds ratio favors the hypothesis, with no credible interval for that probability.

The three approaches described here have different features, and whether these features are advantages or disadvantages will depend on the body of literature and the research question. The quantitizing and the qualitative-as-prior approaches retain quantitative data in their original form (e.g., odds ratios, sample proportions), whereas the qualitizing approach places each quantitative report into a discrete category, potentially resulting in information loss. The quantitizing approach infers numerical information from qualitative data, which is subject to a potentially high degree of uncertainty and may result in information loss from qualitative findings. The qualitizing and qualitative-as-prior approaches use qualitative data in a form closer to that intended by the authors of reports (the presence/absence of statements about certain findings).

Although the qualitative-as-prior approach remains most true to the original form of both the qualitative and quantitative data, the fact that the qualitative data are incorporated into the prior and the quantitative into the posterior means that the method does not inherently treat quantitative and qualitative data with equal weight. The quantitizing approach treats every participant (whether in a qualitative or quantitative study) with equal weight, with the effect that reports based on more participants contribute more evidence to the results. The qualitizing approach treats each report (qualitative or quantitative) with equal weight, regardless of sample size. Either of these characteristics may be a strength or limitation, depending on the researchers' assessments of what will constitute meaningful research synthesis results. The qualitiative-as-prior used both report- and subject-level synthesis; treating each qualitative report with equal weight (in construction of the prior probability) but accounting for the number of participants in synthesizing the quantitative reports.

The choice of whether to treat each report as a single case or to synthesize on the individual level affects the researcher's options for the statistical model. A random effects model, common in research synthesis, requires the assumption of within-report variability and is inappropriate for findings synthesized at the report level. The qualitizing approach uses a random-effects model (although a fixed effects model could be used). The quantitizing approach, with no individual-level data, must use a fixed-effects model. The qualitative-as-prior approach uses a fixed-effects model for the quantitative studies, although it could certainly be adapted to use a random-effects model.

The applicability of Bayesian methods for mixed research synthesis has been demonstrated but is yet to have widespread use. The main limitations include the mathematical background and level of computational skill required to create the Bayesian models and obtain the necessary information about the posterior distribution, the lack of widely-available software to do so, and the difficulty of communicating technically complex methods transparently to a general audience (Sutton & Abrams 2001; Dixon-Woods *et al.* 2004). Once a researcher has attained the required level of expertise, the flexibility of the Bayesian approach to blend different types of information is extremely useful. This inherent flexibility stems directly from the underlying conceptualization of Bayesian probability; that probability can be used to describe uncertainty about population characteristics as well as the randomness associated with sampling and measurement.

We have focused on the two major decisions leading to distinctions between the approaches: the form of the data (qualitizing, quantitizing, or neither) and the choice about which data to include in the prior or likelihood. We have also discussed some of the smaller modeling decisions: for example, the use of a non-informative prior distribution in the quantitizing method, missing data methods to compensate for lack of data in the qualitizing method, and use of qualitative reports alone instead of an expert panel in the qualitative-as-prior method. Any of these decisions could have been made differently. In the application of these Bayesian approaches to mixed research synthesis, it is less important to follow these methods exactly as described here than it is to consider modeling decisions in light of the available data and the research question. Each research synthesis will require its own approach, deviating in ways large or small from those presented here.

Acknowledgments

This article was supported by a National Institute of Nursing Research, National Institutes of Health (5R01NR004907, June 3, 2005–March 31, 2010) grant ("Integrating qualitative and quantitative research findings"), and with resources and facilities at the Veterans Affairs Medical Center in Durham, NC. Views expressed in this article are those of the authors and do not necessarily represent the Department of Veterans Affairs. This chapter draws from information previously presented in papers by Crandell *et al.* (in press) and Voils *et al.* (2009).

References

Abel E, Painter L. (2003) Factors that influence adherence to HIV medications: Perceptions of women and health care providers. *J Assoc Nurses AIDS Care.* **14**(4): 61–9.

Chang Y, Voils CI, Sandelowski M, Hasselblad V, Crandell, JL. (2009) Transforming verbal counts in reports of qualitative descriptive studies into numbers. *Western Journal of Nursing Research.* **31**: 837–852.

Crandell J, Voils CI, Chang Y, Sandelowski M. (In press) Bayesian data augmentation methods for the synthesis of qualitative and quantitative research findings. *Journal of Quality and Quantity.*

Dixon-Woods M, Agarwal S, Young B, Sutton, A. (2004) Integrative approaches to qualitative and quantitative evidence. London: NHS Health Development Agency.

Douglass JL, Sowell RL, Phillips KD. (2003) Using Peplau's theory to examine the psychosocial factors associated with HIV-infected women's difficulty in taking their medications. *J Theory Constr Test.* **7**(1): 10–7.

Durante AJ, Bova CA, Fennie KP, Danvers KA, Holness DR, Burgess JD, *et al.* (2003) Home-based study of anti-HIV drug regimen adherence among HIV-infected women: feasibility and preliminary results. *AIDS Care.* **15**(1): 103–115.

Edwards LV. (2006) Perceived social support and HIV/AIDS medication adherence among African American women. *Qual Health Res.* **16**(5): 679–691.

Gant LM, Welch LA. (2004) Voices less heard: HIV-positive African American women, medication adherence, sexual abuse, and self-care. *J HIV AIDS Soc Serv.* **3**(2): 67–91.

Gelman A, Carlin JB, Stern HS, Rubin DB. (2004) Bayesian Data Analysis (2nd ed). Boca Raton, Florida: Chapman and Hall/CRC.

Hartley H. (1961) The modified Gauss Newton method for the fitting of nonlinear regression functions by least squares. *Technometrics.* **3**: 269–280.

Howard AA, Arnsten JH, Lo Y, Vlahov D, Rich JD, Schuman P, *et al.* (2002) A prospective study of adherence and viral load in a large multi-center cohort of HIV-infected women. *AIDS.* **16**(16): 2175–2182.

Jones, DR, Dixon-Woods, M, Abrams, K, Fitzpatrick, R. (2005) Meta-analysis of qualitative and quantitative evidence: Full report of research activities and results (ESRC ALCD 2 programme) – Available by searching the ESRC social sciences repository. http://www. esrcsocietytoday.ac.uk. Cited 6 January, 2009.

Kalichman SC, Rompa D, DiFonzo K, Simpson D, Austin J, Luke W, *et al.* (2001) HIV treatment adherence in women living with HIV/AIDS: Research based on the Information-Motivation-Behavioral Skills model of health behavior. *J Assoc Nurses AIDS Care.* **12**(4): 58–67.

Kleinman J. (1973) Proportions with extraneous variance: Single and independent samples. *J Am Stat Assoc.* **68**: 46–54.

Lilford RJ, Braunholtz D. (2003) Reconciling the quantitative and qualitative traditions - The Bayesian approach. *Public Money and Management.* **23**: 203–208.

Little RJA, Rubin DB. (2002) Statistical Analysis with Missing Data (2nd ed). Hoboken, New Jersey: John Wiley and Sons.

Liu H, Longshore D, Williams JK, Rivkin I, Loeb T, Warda US, *et al.* (2006) Substance abuse and medication adherence among HIV-positive women with histories of child sexual abuse. *AIDS Behav.* **10**(3): 279–286.

Misener TR, Sowell RL. (1998) HIV-infected women's decisions to take antiretrovirals. *West J Nurs Res.* **20**(4): 431–447.

Mostashari F, Riley E, Selwyn PA, Altice FL. (1998) Acceptance and adherence with antiretroviral therapy among HIV-infected women in a correctional facility. *J Acquir Immune Defic Syndr Hum Retrovirol.* **18**(4): 341–348.

Murphy DA, Greenwell L, Hoffman D. (2002) Factors associated with antiretroviral adherence among HIV-infected women with children. *Women Health.* **36**(1): 97–111.

Phillips KD, Moneyham L, Murdaugh C, Boyd MR, Tavakoli A, Jackson K, *et al.* (2005) Sleep disturbance and depression as barriers to adherence. *Clin Nurs Res.* **14**(3): 273–293.

Pope C, Mays N, Popay J. (2007) Synthesizing Qualitative and Quantitative Health Evidence. Berkshire, England: Open University Press.

Remien RH, Hirky AE, Johnson MO, Weinhardt LS, Whittier D, Le GM. (2003) Adherence to medication treatment: A qualitative study of facilitators and barriers among a diverse sample of HIV + men and women in four U. S. cities. *AIDS Behav.* **7**(1): 61–72.

Richter DL, Sowell RL, Pluto DM. (2002) Attitudes toward antiretroviral therapy among African American women. *Am J Health Behav.* **26**(1): 25–33.

Roberts K, Dixon-Woods M, Fitzpatrick R, Abrams K, Jones DR. (2002) Factors affecting uptake of childhood immunisation: an example of Bayesian synthesis of qualitative and quantitative evidence. *The Lancet.* **360**: 1596–1599.

Roberts KJ, Mann T. (2000) Barriers to antiretroviral medication adherence in HIV-infected women. *AIDS Care.* **12**(4): 377–86.

Sandelowski M, Barroso J. (2007) Handbook for Synthesizing Qualitative Research. New York: Springer.

Schrimshaw EW, Siegel K, Lekas H. (2005) Changes in attitudes toward antiviral medication: A comparison of women living with HIV/AIDS in the pre-HAART and HAART eras. *AIDS Behav.* **9**(3): 267–279.

Schuman P, Ohmit SE, Cohen M, Sacks HS, Richardson J, Young M, *et al.* (2001) Prescription of and adherence to antiretroviral therapy among women with AIDS. *AIDS Behav.* **5**(4): 371–378.

Siegel K, Gorey E. (1997) HIV-infected women: Barriers to AZT use. *Soc Sci Med.* **45**(1): 15–22.

Siegel K, Lekas H, Schrimshaw EW, Johnson JK. Factors associated with HIV-infected women's use or intention to use AZT during pregnancy. *AIDS Educ Prev.* **13**(3): 189–206.

Sowell RL, Phillips KD, Seals BF, Misener TR, Rush C. (2001) HIV-infected women's experiences and beliefs related to AZT therapy during pregnancy. *AIDS Patient Care STDS.* **15**(4): 201–9.

Stone VE, Hogan JW, Schuman P, Rompalo AM, Howard AA, Korkontzelou C, *et al.* (2001) Antiretroviral regimen complexity, self-reported adherence, and HIV patients' understanding of their regimens: Survey of women in the her study. *J Acquir Immune Defic Syndr.* **28**(2): 124–131.

Sutton AJ, Abrams K. (2001) Bayesian methods in meta-analysis and evidence synthesis. *Stat Methods Med Res.* **10**: 277–303.

Tashakkori A, Teddlie C. (2003) Handbook of Mixed Methods in Social and Behavioral Research. Thousand Oaks, CA: Sage.

Voils CI, Hasselblad V, Chang Y, Crandell JL, Lee EJ, Sandelowski, M. (2009) A Bayesian method for the synthesis of evidence from qualitative and quantitative reports: An example from the literature on antiretroviral medication adherence. *Journal of Health Services Research and Policy.* **14**: 226–233.

Wilson TE, Barron Y, Cohen M, Richardson J, Greenblatt R, Sacks HS, *et al.* (2002) Adherence to antiretroviral therapy and its association with sexual behavior in a national sample of women with human immunodeficiency virus. *Clin Infect Dis.* **34**(4): 529–534.

Wilson TE, Ickovics JR, Fernandez MI, Koenig LJ, Walter E. (2001) Self-reported zidovudine adherence among pregnant women with human immunodeficiency virus infection in four US states. *Am J Obstet Gynecol.* **184**(6): 1235–1240.

Wolfram S. (1996) Mathematica. Champaign, IL.: Wolfram Research, Inc.

Wood SA, Tobias C, McCree J. (2004) Medication adherence for HIV positive women caring for children: in their own words. *AIDS Care.* **16**(7): 909–913.

Chapter 8 **Conclusion**

Dr Nathan Manning, PhD

Kleijnen Systematic Reviews
and The Joanna Briggs Institute,
University of Adelaide, Australia

This chapter begins by arguing that the purpose or desired end product of a review should be the key consideration when choosing between methods for qualitative evidence synthesis (QES). The second half of the chapter engages with the notion that the field of QES is characterized by differences in approach. These differences are located within the epistemological and ontological differences which make up qualitative research and the range of disciplines contributing to QES methods. A discussion of approaches to searching and the use of quality assessment reveals substantial overlap between the methods described in this book.

Introduction

This book has provided the reader with a practical guide to common methods used for the synthesis of qualitative evidence. Written by reviewers, and in several cases pioneers of particular approaches, this is a unique collection that provides insights into conducting reviews according to different methods, along with discussion of methodological and epistemological implications. This chapter will take a step back from the particular methods of synthesis to consider the field of qualitative synthesis more broadly, the continuing issues and future directions for qualitative evidence synthesis. The chapter begins by outlining key considerations when tackling a qualitative evidence synthesis (QES), before looking at the challenges and future of a field characterized by multiple different approaches to QES.

To begin, it is useful to remind ourselves of some of the things to consider when starting a systematic review. When beginning a review, it is perhaps most important to consider the purpose of the review and the desired outcomes. Being clear about what a particular review should deliver from

Synthesizing Qualitative Research: Choosing the Right Approach, First Edition.
Edited by Karin Hannes and Craig Lockwood.
© 2012 John Wiley & Sons, Ltd. Published 2012 by John Wiley & Sons, Ltd.

the outset will make supplementary work and decisions much more straight-forward. One needs to choose a review method that can provide the desired outcomes. For example, if the purpose of a review is to generate a conceptual model then choosing an approach like meta-aggregation, discussed by Hannes and Pearson, which is designed to provide clear, practical advice to clinicians/practitioners may not be the ideal choice. Deciding on what a review is to deliver should be the key consideration in choosing a review method. From here, we can see how later work and decisions are aided by this early clarity.

Each of the methods discussed in this collection have been designed for the synthesis of primary studies, in contrast to basic methods like grounded theory (Glaser & Strauss 1967), which have been adapted for qualitative evidence synthesis. For six qualitative evidence synthesis specific methods discussed in this book, a clear question is very useful in setting some parameters around the research. This does not mean the question need be fixed in stone, but all research must begin somewhere and a clear question will help guide and focus the review.

Knowing what the review is to deliver *and* the review question, there are several other considerations to keep in mind when choosing a method, but determining which method suits your needs is made easier by this prepa-ratory work. For example, deciding whether to use a review method that can synthesize both qualitative *and* quantitative evidence or only qualitative data is a question that relates directly to the desired output of the review and the review question. If the key purpose of a review is to theorize or conceptualize, and the review question relates to men's experiences of undergoing vasectomy, then quantitative evidence is likely of less relevance. However, for a review undertaken to inform clinical practice looking at effective interventions to increase breastfeeding, bringing together effec-tiveness data from quantitative studies and qualitative data regarding women's experience of breastfeeding and the particular interventions and their delivery/implementation would produce a strong foundation from which to make recommendations for practice.

Finally, when deciding on a particular method of qualitative evidence synthesis, reviewers will need to think about the experience and expertise of their team along with the available resources. Choosing a highly interpretive approach like critical interpretive synthesis (CIS) when it does not match up with the experience mix or epistemological stance of the team is setting the project up for serious challenges if not failure. Having a clear notion of what the review is to deliver, and being mindful of the kind of review that the review team is capable of producing with the resources and expertise available, is crucial for ensuring a project's success.

Table 8.1 Select features of qualitative evidence synthesis methods

Synthesis method	Epistemology	Type of data	End product
Bayesian synthesis	More realist	Qualitative & quantitative	Statistical model
Critical interpretive synthesis	More idealist	Qualitative & quantitative	Conceptual model/theory
Meta-aggregation	More realist	Qualitative	Recommendations for practitioners/policy
Meta-ethnography	More idealist	Qualitative	Conceptual model/theory
Mixed methods synthesis	More realist	Qualitative & quantitative	Recommendations for policy & practice
Realist synthesis	More realist	Qualitative & quantitative	Theory & recommendations for policy

Table 8.1 above provides an overly schematic breakdown of the different approaches to qualitative evidence synthesis. The table borrows Kavanagh *et al.*'s (Chapter 6) notion of a realist–idealist continuum to provide an indication of a method's epistemological grounding. While we should encourage reviewers to try different methods of synthesis, it is prudent to ensure some level of overlap between the general epistemological stance of the review team and the chosen synthesis method. Given the dominance of the scientific method in all walks of life, many may be more familiar with realist/positivist epistemologies, and hence considering the epistemology of a review method may be particularly consequential when entertaining a more idealist or interpretive approach.

Consideration of the type of data to be synthesized is a less contentious matter, but just as important for ensuring the review provides the required outcomes and can answer the review question(s).

Finally, the table points to the end product the method is designed to produce. This is no doubt an oversimplification – most reviews will discuss implications for practice and research. Moreover, synthesis methods designed to inform practice have been used in model/theory development (Briggs & Flemming 2007). Nonetheless, it remains the case that some review methods lend themselves more to recommendations for practice/policy while others are more suited to theory/model development. Putting simplifications to one side, the desired end product of the review and considerations of type of data and epistemology are key considerations for a team planning to undertake a review involving qualitative evidence synthesis.

Beset by questions and alternatives

Qualitative evidence synthesis is sometimes characterized as a field defined by a range of differences. There are different approaches to using review protocols and developing a review question; the review question can be a guiding tool which is revisited and revised in an iterative fashion as the review progresses or clearly defined at the beginning of the review and used to anchor the project. There are different ways of searching the literature; some aim to be exhaustive while others use sampling techniques. Some methods use quality assessment as a standard step in the review process while others do not. Some undertake quality assessment but do not use it as grounds to exclude poor quality papers. Some approaches can synthesize qualitative *and* quantitative data while others can only work with qualitative research. Some methods integrate qualitative and quantitative syntheses while others keep them separate. When it comes to analysis some methods limit the scope for reviewer interpretation of the data while a high level of interpretation is intrinsic to other methods. Finally, some methods lend themselves more to theoretical and model development while others are more suited to informing practice and policy.

Unfortunately, for those seeking simple answers, there are yet further differences between these methods, differences that transcend the actual method or recipe for doing a qualitative evidence synthesis. These are fundamental differences that relate to the epistemological and ontological foundations of particular review methods. Is there ultimately a "real" world that researchers should be striving to describe in the face of partial and imperfect knowledge or is the only knowledge we have access to interpretation? How does our way of knowing the world relate to our understanding of human subjectivity? Is social life dynamic and made up of reflexive social actors actively engaged in creating their worlds or is it flatter and more uniform than that? These questions point to the different disciplines and traditions of inquiry from which particular qualitative evidence synthesis methods have emerged (for a general discussion of epistemology and ontology in qualitative research, see Denzin and Lincoln 2008). As a result, qualitative evidence synthesis is not a unified field. It represents a variety of epistemological positions and has been developed in several academic disciplines. This has made it difficult to speak in one voice – the desirability of the field being univocal is discussed below.

The field of qualitative evidence synthesis may look disordered when viewed from the perspective of traditional systematic reviews using meta-analysis. Such methods are now established across healthcare disciplines with very clear and detailed descriptions of the methods (Centre for Reviews and

Dissemination 2009; Higgins & Green 2009). But we would do well to remember that notions of evidence-based medicine (EBM) and healthcare, which promoted traditional systematic reviews, initially faced serious and sustained criticism (Charlton 1997; Sackett *et al.* 1996). More fundamentally, those working with traditional systematic reviews, and even new review areas like diagnostics (Leeflang *et al.* 2008; Whiting *et al.* 2003), generally operate within the same realist/positivist or post-positivist epistemology. This means there is considerable common ground which does not need to be questioned and the business of how to do reviews can be got on with.

Working within a field characterized by different epistemologies can mean sharing less common ground. However, rather than the range of different approaches to qualitative evidence synthesis being cause for concern they should be understood as reflecting the vigor of the field and the diverse roots of qualitative inquiry. The range of qualitative methodologies and methods used in primary research were developed in attempts to engage with the social world in all its complexity. Modernity and social life are dynamic and as such primary researchers have employed a range of methodologies and methods in their attempts to understand, interpret and change the world around them.

The range of qualitative evidence synthesis methods available may make the field more confusing to outsiders, but this breadth is much more a benefit than a cost. At a practical level, considerations about the review question, the team's experience mix, and the desired outcome of the review will significantly cut down the range of qualitative evidence synthesis methods applicable to any given review.

In recent years various critics have argued that the evidence-based movement is part of a drive to set boundaries on valid knowledge and discount all knowledge produced outside realist/positivist or post-positivist paradigms (Denzin 2009; Holmes *et al.* 2006; Willis & White 2002). These critics selectively draw upon the evidence-based movement in healthcare and education to argue that the movement has created a hierarchy of knowledge where only some forms of knowledge count. One means of challenging these critics is by providing a fuller description of the field of evidence-based healthcare, which sharply contrasts with the emaciated, "RCT-only" view typically constructed by these authors (see Holmes 2006; Pearson 2006). A further clear indication that such "totalitarianism" is not taking place within qualitative evidence synthesis is a book such as this, which describes several methods for conducting qualitative synthesis at differing stages of development and from across the realist–idealist continuum. If proponents of qualitative evidence synthesis were calling for one method of synthesis in all circumstances, this indeed, would be cause for concern.

Continuing controversies?

Before turning to a discussion of the debate *between* methods of qualitative evidence synthesis, it is worth briefly considering the notion that combining qualitative studies in such a synthesis is anathema to the particularistic nature of qualitative research itself. The idea being that qualitative studies are a unique interaction of the researcher(s) and participant(s) in a particular social context at a particular moment of time. As such the findings may relate only to those particular participants in that particular social context and historical moment and the researcher(s) interpretations. This being the case it makes little sense to combine such particularistic studies, which by their nature do not provide findings that might be translated to different participants, social contexts, and researchers. This problem can be countered in a number of ways (Sandelowski 1996). There are responses from either end of the realist–idealist continuum. If one adopts a more realist position and accepts that while knowledge is partial and imperfect, researchers are in fact aiming to understand an underlying social reality, then one can draw upon qualitative research to inform policy and practice if mindful of the particularities of qualitative studies. From a more idealist perspective, qualitative inquiry is a hermeneutic process where the primary goal is interpretation and explanation of the social world. From this position, qualitative studies can be drawn upon in the interest of furthering our knowledge and understanding of the social world.

Beyond the challenge of a field characterized by a range of methods for qualitative evidence synthesis, these different methods have also spawned a number of key differences about the review process itself. The discussion below focuses on approaches to searching and study selection and appraising the literature.

Searching and study selection – comprehensive or sample?

In traditional quantitative systematic reviews a structured search strategy is developed for relevant databases with the aim of collecting all relevant research for a given review question. This approach loosely reflects the sampling ideal of a positivist/post-positivist paradigm – collect a sample large enough such that one can have a high level of confidence in generalizing from the sample to the general population. Similarly, reviewers want access to as many relevant studies as possible so they can make an accurate and valid assessment of effectiveness for a given question. Indeed, some argue that qualitative reviews should also aim to include all possible studies (see Barroso *et al.* 2003; Walsh & Downe 2005). In contrast, primary qualitative research typically uses much smaller samples and rarely aims to make generalizations from a sample to the population at large. Qualitative researchers tend to focus on "thick description" (Geertz 1973), gaining an in-depth understanding of a given phenomena and its social context, which typically means the research methods are time intensive. Various sampling techniques have been developed to meet the needs of qualitative researchers (Pope & Mays 2006). Given the emphasis on understanding and interpretation of the social world and the unique sampling methods of qualitative research, some have argued qualitative evidence synthesis should borrow sampling techniques from qualitative primary research (Booth 2001).

The reader will recall that there were differences in the approach to study selection among the six review methods discussed in this book. Meta-aggregation, meta-ethnography, mixed methods, and critical interpretive synthesis included all relevant papers identified. However, other examples of CIS have used sampling (Dixon-Woods *et al.* 2006). The realist review recommends using saturation to construct a sample of papers for review, but Wong also notes the benefit of going through all 249 papers. Therefore, most of the methods described in this book aim to be comprehensive in their approach to searching and selecting studies for synthesis.

A further advantage of a comprehensive search and approach to study selection is the more complete view of the literature this yields. Systematic reviews are not just about gaining new insights from the pooling and interpretation of two or more studies; they should also be part of a process which informs primary research. A more comprehensive approach to searching and study selection furnishes a review with a strong platform from which to make comment about a given research field, its methodological strengths and weaknesses, and where gaps in the literature exist.

Quality assessment

Evaluating the quality of studies is a typical step in traditional systematic reviews. It is primarily used to assess the internal validity of included studies and exclude research with an unacceptable risk of bias, thereby ensuring the rigor of the review's findings. However, the application and relevance of quality assessment for qualitative systematic reviews is contested (Dixon-Woods *et al.* 2004). To a greater or lesser extent all qualitative syntheses, regardless of method used, are interpretive exercises aimed at gaining an understanding of a particular phenomenon. As such, perhaps the ultimate criteria by which a piece of research should be judged is its ability to contribute to that understanding. It is most unlikely that poor quality research will provide unique insights into a given phenomena, but it is possible (Harden 2008). Nonetheless, we all undertake some form of quality assessment as readers of research, and evaluating study quality as part of systematic reviews will likely lead to improvements in the *reporting* of primary qualitative research (Sandelowski & Barosso 2002), if not the research itself. If quality assessment is to be done, it should be fully reported for the sake of transparency and as a means of informing future primary research.

In this book, most of the methods outlined – meta-ethnography, meta-aggregation, mixed methods, and critical interpretive synthesis – explicitly discuss the use of checklists to appraise a study's quality. The realist review takes a different tack asking the reviewer to assess not an entire study but the rigor of a relevant piece of data. Nonetheless the question remains as to which appraisal checklist one should use. There are a vast number of checklists (Spencer *et al.* 2003) and little work has been done to evaluate these tools (Dixon-Woods *et al.* 2007; Hannes *et al.* 2010). A synthesis method may include an assessment tool as part of its approach, like the meta-aggregation described by Hannes and Pearson. When this is not the case, as for most methods, thinking about the review team's experience with qualitative research will be instructive. A review team with little experience of qualitative research may opt to choose a checklist which provides relatively detailed explanations of each quality item, while a more experienced team will likely need less guidance on such issues and could opt for a checklist that does well in evaluating the intrinsic methodological quality of an original study (Hannes *et al.* 2010).

This discussion of study selection and quality assessment has highlighted the similarity between the synthesis methods described in this book. Clearly there are important differences between approaches, particularly with regard to epistemology, method of synthesis, and review output. However, when we look at the review process – at least for the six methods described in this book – there is greater overlap than is usually acknowledged. While the field of qualitative evidence synthesis does not offer one prescriptive method for the synthesis of qualitative research, there is significant agreement across the methods on many key steps of a review.

Review questions are critically important for all methods – regardless of whether the question is fixed from the outset or remains flexible as the research progresses. Some approaches set a review question at the beginning of a review while others iteratively develop a question with the literature. Most methods advocate using a range of searching techniques as identifying qualitative research can be difficult (Greenhalgh & Peacock 2005). A comprehensive approach to searching and study selection is taken by most methods, while sampling and data saturation can be useful for CIS and realist synthesis. Quality assessment is generally accepted and the use of checklists is recommended. Methods for data synthesis vary but this reflects the different epistemological traditions of qualitative research rather than any incoherence on behalf of the field. The range of analysis methods also provides reviewers with flexibility when choosing a review method.

Concluding remarks

Finally, it is worth considering what the future may hold for qualitative evidence synthesis. While some synthesis methods have now been with us for decades (Noblit & Hare 1988), it was really the past decade that witnessed the renaissance of methods for qualitative evidence synthesis. This revival began in healthcare, but qualitative research is now being synthesized and applied in a growing number of fields – for example, social work, law, and education. And this will likely expand as governments increasingly call for public policy to be informed by evidence. As reviewers we are now well placed to meet this demand with a range of different approaches to qualitative evidence synthesis able to answer a variety of review questions and provide different kinds of outcomes. Mixed method reviews and using QES to add value to traditional effectiveness reviews will also be important sites for methodological development. Stand alone qualitative reviews will continue to be important but qualitative research also has much to offer in enhancing the delivery, uptake, and implementation of interventions known to be effective. May the following decades see the consolidation of established synthesis methods, the ongoing development of new methods to meet emerging challenges, and the growth of qualitative systematic reviewers from a variety of epistemological, methodological and disciplinary backgrounds.

References

Barroso J, Gollop, CJ, Sandelowski, M, Meynell, J, Pearce, PF, Collins, LJ. (2003) The challenges of searching for and retrieving qualitative studies. *Western Journal of Nursing Research.* 25: 153–178.

Booth A. (2001) Cochrane or cock-eyed? How should we conduct systematic reviews of qualitative research? In Qualitative evidence-based conference: Taking a critical stance Coventry University 2001. Available at: http://www.leeds.ac.uk/educol/documents/00001724.htm [accessed 7 June 2011].

Briggs M., Flemming K. (2007) Living with leg ulceration: a synthesis of qualitative research. *Journal of Advanced Nursing.* 59(4): 319–328.

Centre for Reviews and Dissemination (CRD) (2009) CRD's guidance for undertaking reviews in health care. York CRD, University of York.

Charlton BG. (1997) Restoring the balance: evidence-based medicine put in its place. *J Eval Clin Pract.* 3: 87–98.

Critical Appraisal Skills Programme, (CASP), (2006) 10 questions to help you make sense of qualitative research. http://www.sph.nhs.uk/sph-files/casp-appraisal-tools/Qualitative%20Appraisal%20Tool.pdf [accessed 7 June 2011].

Denzin N. (2009) The elephant in the living room: or extending the conversation about the politics of evidence. *Qualitative Research.* 9(2): 139–160.

Denzin N, Lincoln Y. (eds.) (2008) *The Landscape of Qualitative Research* (3rd Ed). Thousand Oaks: Sage Publications, Inc.

Dixon-Woods, M. Shaw, R. L. Agarwal, S. Smith, J. A. (2004) The problem of appraising qualitative research. *Quality & Safety in Health Care.* 13: 223–225.

Dixon-Woods M, Cavers D, Agarwal S, Annandale E, Arthur A, Harvey J, Hsu R. Katbama S, Olsen R, Smith L, Riley R, Sutton AJ. (2006) Conducting a critical interpretive synthesis on the literature on access to healthcare by vulnerable groups. *BMC Medical Research Methodology.* 6: 35.

Dixon-Woods, M. Sutton, A. Shaw, R. Miller, T. Smith, J. Young, B. Bonas, S. Booth, A. Jones, D. (2007) Appraising qualitative research for inclusion in systematic reviews: a quantitative and qualitative comparison of three methods. *Journal of Health Services Research and Policy.* 12: 42–47.

Geertz, C. (1973) *The Interpretation of Cultures: Selected Essays.* New York: Basic Books.

Glaser, BG, Strauss, AL. (1967) *The Discovery of Grounded Theory: Strategies for Qualitative Research.* Chicago: Aldine Publishing.

Greenhalgh T, Peacock R. (2005) Effectiveness and efficiency of search methods in systematic reviews of complex evidence: audit of primary sources. *BMJ.* 5: 331 (7524): 1064–5.

Hannes K, Lockwood C, Pearson A. (2010) A comparative analysis of three online appraisal instruments' ability to assess validity in qualitative research. *Qual Health Res.* 20(12): 1736–43.

Harden, Angela (2008) Critical appraisal and qualitative research: exploring sensitivity analysis. In: *NCRM Research Methods Festival 2008, 30th June – 3rd July 2008,* St Catherine's College, Oxford.

Higgins JPT, Green S(Eds). (2009) Cochrane Handbook for Systematic Reviews of Interventions Version 5.0.2 (updated September 2009). The Cochrane Collaboration, 2009. Available from www.cochrane-handbook.org [accessed 7 June 2011].

Holmes C. (2006) Never mind the evidence, feel the width: a response to Holmes, Murray, Perron and Rail. *International Journal of Evidence-Based Healthcare.* 4(3): 187–188.

Holmes D, Murray SJ, Perron A, Rail G. (2006) Deconstructing the evidence-based discourse in health sciences: truth, power and fascism. *International Journal of Evidence Based Healthcare.* 4(3): 180–186.

Leeflang MM, Debets-Ossenkopp YJ, Visser CE, Scholten RJPM, Hooft L, Bijlmer HA, Reitsma JB, Bossuyt PMM, Vandenbroucke-Grauls CM. (2008) Galactomannan detection for invasive aspergillosis in immunocompromised patients. *Cochrane Database of Systematic Reviews.* Issue 4. Art. No.: CD007394. DOI: 10.1002/14651858.CD007394.

Noyes J, Popay J, Pearson A, Hannes K, Booth A. (2009) Qualitative research and Cochrane reviews. In: Higgins JPT, Green S. (Eds), *Cochrane Handbook for Systematic Reviews of Interventions Version 5.0.1* (updated September 2008), chapter 20. The Cochrane Collaboration. Available from www.cochrane-handbook.org [accessed 7 June 2011].

Pearson A. (2006) Scientists, postmodernists or fascists? *International Journal of Evidence-Based Healthcare.* 4(4): 385–391.

Pope C, Mays N. (Eds) (2006) *Qualitative Research in Health Care.* 3rd ed. Blackwell Publishing: Oxford.

Sackett D, Rosenberg WMC, Gray JAM, Haynes RB, Richardson WS. (1996) Evidence based medicine: what it is and what it isn't. *BMJ.* 312: 71.

Sandelowski M., Barosso J. (2002) Reading qualitative studies. *International Journal of Qualitative Methods.* 1(1): 74–108.

Sandelowski M. (1996) One is the liveliest number: The case orientation of qualitative research. *Research in Nursing & Health.* **19**: 525–529.

Spencer L, Ritchie J, Lewis J, *et al.* (2003) Quality in qualitative evaluation: a framework for assessing research evidence. Government Chief Social Researcher's Office, Occasional Series; No 2.

Walsh D., Downe S. (2005) Meta-synthesis method for qualitative research: a literature review. *Journal of Advanced Nursing.* **50**(2): 204–211.

Whiting P, Rutjes AWS, Reitsma JB, Bossuyt PMM, Kleijnen J. (2003) The development of QUADAS: a tool for the quality assessment of studies of diagnostic accuracy included in systematic reviews. *BMC Medical Research Methodology.* **3**: 25.

Willis, E., White, Kevin (2002) Positivism resurgent: the epistemological foundations of evidence-based medicine. *Health Sociology Review.* **11**(2): 5–15.

Index

Notes: Page numbers in *italics* refer to Figures; those in **bold** to Tables. Abbreviations: CIS = critical interpretive syntheses; EBP = evidence-based practice.

Adams B., 87
Adams S., 46, 47, *48*, 49–53, 54, 56
adherence see medicine taking
agency, realist reviews, 83–4, 87–9, 94, 108, 110–11
aggregative syntheses, 5–6, **14**, 22–3
see also meta-aggregation worked example; thematic analysis
Amir Z., 9
Anderson R., 84
antiretroviral medication adherence, 141–57
appraisal of studies
checklists, 71, **72**, 168
controversies, 27, 167–8
critical interpretive syntheses, 71–2
meta-aggregation, 27
meta-ethnography, 45–6, 55–6
mixed method syntheses, 126–9
realist reviews, 97, 105–6, 168
asthma, medicine taking for, 44–56
Atlas-Ti software, 72, 76

Barnett-Page E., 116
Barroso J., 7
Bayes' rule, 140

Bayesian meta-analysis, 6, 9, **14**
qualitative and quantitative data see Bayesian syntheses
Bayesian statistical framework
likelihood, 139, 140
mixed research syntheses, 140–1
posterior distribution, 140
prior distribution, 139, 140
probability, 138–9, 140
Bayesian syntheses, 137–57
Bayesian statistical framework, 138–41
definition, **14**
limitations, 156
qualitative-as-prior, 141, 149–57
qualitizing, 141, 146–9, 150, 152–7
quantitizing, 141–6, 152–7
question formulation, 141
Bélanger E., 7
Belgian healthcare, barriers to EBP, 21–37
beliefs, medicine taking, 44–56
Benbasat I., 103
bias, assessing risk of, 126
Braunholtz D., 149–50
Buston K., 46, 47, *48*, 49–53, 54

Synthesizing Qualitative Research: Choosing the Right Approach, First Edition.
Edited by Karin Hannes and Craig Lockwood.
© 2012 John Wiley & Sons, Ltd. Published 2012 by John Wiley & Sons, Ltd.

Lightning Source UK Ltd.
Milton Keynes UK
UKHW022209180220
358954UK00002B/2